Pregnancy and Fluoride Do Not Mix

Prenatal Fluoride and
Premature Birth
Preeclampsia
Autism

John Douglas MacArthur, Jr.

For Jenanurse
w/ thanks

John

Pregnancy and Fluoride Do Not Mix

Prenatal Fluoride and
Premature Birth
Preeclampsia
Autism

John Douglas MacArthur, Jr.

©2016

Updated September 2018

ISBN-10: 1512230227
ISBN-13: 978-1512230222

CreateSpace Independent
Publishing Platform

Back cover illustration courtesy
Sheng Yi Lee • ©2015

PregnancyAndFluorideDoNotMix.com

The scientific evidence gathered in this volume
validates the need and right of families
to know the risks of drinking
fluoridated tap water.

Contents

"A long habit of not thinking a thing wrong,
gives it a superficial appearance of being right."

– Thomas Paine (1776)
Common Sense

Introduction

Before focusing on pregnancy and neurodevelopment, I wrote about neurodegeneration. Then I learned that the leading predictor of long-term neurological disabilities in children is premature (preterm) birth. Clinical studies in India had already shown that fluoride is a significant risk factor. This was confirmed by a New York public health study that found community water fluoridation was independently associated with an increased risk of preterm birth.

The US preterm birth rate is unusually high, so my first project was an in-depth review of the connections between maternal fluoride consumption and preterm birth. Next I explored preeclampsia, the poorly understood pregnancy complication with high maternal and infant death rates. Compelling scientific evidence links fluoride and *placental fluorosis* to the pathogenesis of preeclampsia.

The third report published by the *Townsend Letter: The Examiner of Alternative Medicine* presented new research and diverse evidence for how prenatal fluoride impairs neurological and immunological development seen in autism spectrum disorder – including via the gastrointestinal tract – as the National Research Council indicated in 2006: "Fluorides have the ability to interfere with the functions of the brain... by direct and indirect means."

As discussed in Chapter 3, babies in the womb swallow amniotic fluid, whose fluoride levels increase when their mothers consume more fluoride. The strong antimicrobial properties of fluoride can disrupt proper bacterial colonization of the GI tract and adversely affect the developing immune and nervous systems.

Known and Growing Safety Concerns

In 1997, when the safety thresholds of fluoride were established for children, health authorities ignored children in the womb and continue to do so 20 years later, despite increasing and compelling evidence of fluoride's risk to the developing brain.

In 2009, a team of researchers at the EPA's Neurotoxicology Division found *substantial evidence* that fluoride is one of 107 chemicals (page 2) shown to be "toxic to the developing mammalian nervous system." Other "developmental neurotoxicants" on the list with fluoride include substances pregnant women already should avoid: cocaine, ethanol (alcohol), lead, mercury, nicotine, thalidomide.

Building a Database of Developmental Neurotoxicants:
Evidence from Human and Animal Studies

Neurotoxicology Div. U.S. EPA

Chemicals with **Substantial** Evidence of Developmental Neurotoxicity (n≈100)

2-Ethoxyethyl Acetate	Diazepam	Naltrexone
Acibenzolar-S-methyl	Cytosine Arabinoside	Nicotine
Acrylamide	DEET	Methoxyethanol, 2-
Aldicarb	Deltamethrin	Methylazoxymethanol
Allethrin	Diazinon	Methylmercury
Aluminum (cl or lactate)	Dieldrin	Ozone
Amino-nicotinamide(6-)	Diethylstilbestrol	Paraquat
Aminopterin	Diphenylhydantoin	Parathion (ethyl)
Amphetamine(d-)	Epidermal Growth Factor	PBDEs
Arsenic	Ethanol	PCBs (generic)
Aspartame	Ethylene thiourea	Penicillamine
Azacytidine(5-)	Flourouracil(5-)	Permethrin
Benomyl	Fluazinam	Phenylacetate
Benzene	Fluoride	Phenylalanine (d,l)
Bioallethrin	Griseofulvin	Phthalate, di-(2-ethylhexyl)
Bis(tri-n-butyltin)oxide	Haloperidol	Propylthiouracil
Bisphenol A	Halothane	Retinoids/vit.A/isotretinoin
Bromodeoxyuridine(5-)	Heptachlor	Salicylate
Butylated Hydroxy Anisol	Hexachlorobenzene	Tebuconazole
Butylated hydroxytoluene	Hexachlorophene	Tellurium (salts)
Cadmium	Hydroxyurea	Terbutaline
Caffeine	Imminodiproprionitrile (IDPN)	Thalidomide
Carbamazepine	Ketamine	THC
Carbaryl	Lead	Toluene
Carbon monoxide	Lindane	Triamcinolone
Chlordecone	LSD	Tributyltin chloride
Chlordiazepoxide	Maneb	Trichlorfon
Chlorine dioxide	Medroxyprogesterone	Trichloroethylene
Chlorpromazine	Mepivacaine	Triethyllead
Chlorpyrifos	Methadone	Triethyltin
Cocaine	Methanol	Trimethyltin
Colcemid	Methimazole	Trypan blue
Colchicine	Methylparathion	Urethane
Cypermethrin	Monosodium Glutamate	Valproate
Dexamethasone	MPTP	Vincristine
Diamorphine hydrochloride	Naloxone	

In 2015, those researchers said fluoride is one of 22 "gold standard" chemicals "well documented to alter human neurodevelopment."

> "Neurotoxins are most damaging during pregnancy because of the heightened susceptibility of the embryonic and fetal brain to developmental disruption... The nature and severity of that disruption depend... most important, on the timing during the developmental process."
>
> – National Scientific Council on the Developing Child (2009)

In 2017, a well-designed 12-year study funded by the US National Institutes of Health found a strong correlation between fluoride levels currently experienced by pregnant women in the US and lower IQ in their children at ages 4 and 6-12 years old. It was conducted largely by specialists in the field, who had done similar studies on other environmental neurotoxins.

In 2018, they reported that higher maternal fluoride exposure has an adverse impact on cognitive development in the first 3 years of life.

Despite growing evidence of harm from prenatal fluoride exposure, health authorities continue to disregard fetuses, as they did in 1997 when the *Tolerable Upper Intake Level* (UL) of fluoride was determined for children – but not for babies in the womb – whose UL would be "significantly lower." In fluoridated cities today, fetal fluoride *intake levels* are comparable to what their UL is reasonably estimated to be.

When a pregnant woman drinks fluoridated tap water throughout the day, as recommended by health authorities, her 3rd-trimester baby's fluoride *intake level* is higher than a 5-year-old child's who swallows more than a pea-sized dab of fluoride toothpaste, the FDA's "contact poison control" threshold. (See Appendix A.)

Validating these known and emerging safety concerns, the new and diverse scientific evidence presented in this thoroughly documented volume (>300 references, mostly PubMed) details the numerous links between prenatal fluoride exposure and adverse health consequences.

I sincerely hope this information will lead to more children entering the world with vibrant and fully functioning brains.

– John D. MacArthur

This is a Human Rights Issue

It is inexcusable to knowingly and needlessly expose babies in the womb to a developmental neurotoxin every day during the months they are most vulnerable to neurological impairment.

Fluoridated tap water must carry a pregnancy warning.

Chapter 1

A global review of recent laboratory, clinical, and ecological evidence that fluoride is a significant risk factor for premature birth and long-term neurological disabilities in children.

An earlier version of this report was
published in the November 2013 *Townsend Letter:
The Examiner of Alternative Medicine*

Fluoride, Premature Birth and Impaired Neurodevelopment

Premature or preterm birth is birth prior to 37 weeks (8.5 months) of pregnancy. According to the US Institute of Medicine:

> "Those born preterm have an appreciable risk of long-term neurological impairment and developmental delay...

> "Preterm infants are more likely to have lower IQs and require significantly more educational assistance than children who were born at term...

> "The annual societal economic burden associated with preterm birth in the United States was at least $26.2 billion in 2005, or $51,600 per infant born preterm."[1]

Preterm birth is the most common pregnancy complication that can seriously compromise the newborn brain's viability and normal development. Many studies have documented the prevalence of a broad range of neurodevelopmental disabilities and dysfunctions in people who were born preterm, including mental retardation, ADHD, and major depression.

Prenatal Brain Development

The genesis and wiring of the human brain during fetal development is one of the most remarkable feats in all of biology. During the last trimester, dynamic changes occur in the two brain areas most important to cognitive processes: the cerebellum whose surface area increases 30-fold; and the cerebral cortex whose white matter undergoes striking changes.[2]

Premature birth can interrupt this vital developmental process, as British researchers showed using a novel form of magnetic resonance imaging to track the growing complexity of nerve cells in the fetal brain before the normal time of birth. Maturation was most rapid in areas of the cortex relating to social and emotional processing, decision making, working memory, and visual-spatial processing – functions often impaired after premature birth.

> "These findings highlight a key stage of brain development where the neurons branch out to create a complex, mature structure. We can now see that this happens in the latter stages of development that would usually take place in healthy babies when they are still in the womb...

"With this study we found that the earlier a baby is born, the less mature the cortex structure. The weeks a baby loses in the womb really matter." – Centre for the Developing Brain at King's College London[3,4]

US Preterm Birth Rate Unusually High

The misconception that preterm birth is a third-world problem was shattered in May 2012 by the first global report to compare preterm birthrates in 184 countries. Three years in the making, "Born Too Soon: The Global Action Report on Preterm Birth" was produced jointly by the World Health Organization, Save the Children, March of Dimes, and Partnership for Maternal, Newborn and Child Health.[5]

America lags behind 130 other nations in preterm birth rate. The United States is similar to developing countries in the percentage of mothers who give birth before their children are due. "It does worse than any Western European country and considerably worse than Japan or the Scandinavian countries," reported Donald G. McNeil, Jr. in the *New York Times*. Most European countries are in the 7% to 9% range, while the United States shares the 12% range with Kenya, Turkey, Thailand, East Timor, and Honduras – meaning that one in nine births is early.[6]

"This report offers conclusive evidence that the United States rate of preterm birth has been far too high for far too long," says March of Dimes president Dr. Jennifer Howse. "We have failed to do enough to prevent preterm births and help more mothers carry their babies full-term."[7]

"If somebody had a simple explanation of why the UK and Europe do much better, I wouldn't believe them," says preterm birth expert Dr. Gordon C. S. Smith. "The reality is, for most preterm births, we just don't understand the cause."[6]

Residence in the US a Risk Factor for Preterm Birth

A 2012 study involving 2,141 women revealed that duration of stay in the US is associated with increased risk of preterm birth for Hispanic women. Dr. Radek K. Bukowski, an expert on premature birth at the University of Texas Medical Branch in Galveston, found that the longer a woman lived in this country, the greater her chances of giving birth prematurely.

Women living in the US for less than 10 years had a 3.4% frequency of preterm birth. Those here for 10+ years had a 7.4% frequency. Women born in the US had a 10% frequency of preterm birth.[8]

The findings support the hypothesis that preterm birth is, at least in part, related to environmental, potentially preventable, factors. It remains unclear what specific environmental factors protect or predispose women to preterm birth. Even after controlling for risk factors such as age, poverty, smoking, obesity, and diabetes, Bukowski admitted: "We really don't have an explanation for what's behind it. It's something they acquire here."[6]

Best-Available Science Will Reduce Preterm Birth by Only 5%

Although preterm birth is the leading cause of death for children younger than five years in high-income countries, second leading cause worldwide, and a major contributor to the "global burden of disease," it wasn't until 2013 that the first multi-country analysis of trends in preterm birth rates was published.

The international team of researchers concluded, "The current potential for preterm birth prevention is shockingly small." If five proven interventions were implemented, it would lower the preterm rate from an average 9.6% of live births to 9.1%. The most effective of these evidence-based interventions is decreasing non-medically indicated caesarean deliveries and induced labor. Dr. Joy Lawn of Save the Children, who coordinated the research, says, "The best-available science will allow just 5 percent relative reduction in high-income countries' preterm birth rates by 2015." Note: of the 39 countries with a "very high human development index," the US has the third highest preterm birth rate (after Cyprus and Bahrain).[9,10]

Because the triggers for premature labor are not fully understood, the poor performance by the US is partly a mystery, said Dr. Alan E. Guttmacher, Director of the National Institute of Child Health and Human Development. "This underscores the need for more research," especially because, as the March of Dimes points out, in up to 40% of cases, the cause of preterm birth is unknown.

It also underscores the need to acknowledge existing research: laboratory, clinical, and ecological evidence that fluoride consumption is a significant risk factor for preterm birth – as this report documents. Unfortunately, health agencies and organizations in the United States typically ignore such research.

Fluoride: Ancient Enemy of Biological Systems

Many Americans think there's nothing wrong with fluoride, a chemical added to nearly three-fourths of their public water supplies and now permeates the nation's processed food and beverage chain.

Even Ronald R. Breaker, PhD, a National Academy of Sciences award-winning molecular biologist with a doctorate in biochemistry "did not know that biology cared much about this ion."[11]

Breaker and his team of experts in microbiology and bioinformatics at Yale University's Howard Hughes Medical Institute study a type of noncoding RNA called a *riboswitch* that helps turn genes on and off. In 2011, they discovered a new riboswitch but could not figure out its function, until a chemistry graduate student "overcame any biases" and quickly demonstrated that pure fluoride indeed triggers riboswitch function that helps cells fight fluoride's "antimicrobial properties."[11-13]

"Despite this evidence, we were still unwilling to accept that fluoride was the natural target," admits Breaker. "It is very likely no one would have solved the mystery of fluoride riboswitches for several more decades, if we had not been lucky enough to receive a contaminated chemical sample spiked with fluoride."[11]

Genes associated with fluoride-sensitive riboswitches are very widespread in biology. Breaker said this new riboswitch is "one of the only non-coding RNAs we've ever found that's present in both bacteria and archaea," a recently identified major domain of life. This suggests an ancient biological system that cells have evolved to deal with fluoride's toxicity.[13,14]

Molecular Mechanisms of Fluoride Toxicity
The authors of a comprehensive 2010 scientific review note that until the 1990s, the toxicity of fluoride was largely ignored due to its "good reputation" for preventing dental caries via topical application in toothpastes. In the last decade, however, interest in its undesirable effects has resurfaced due to the awareness that "this element interacts with cellular systems even at low doses."[15]

> "Even though some studies report no clear evidence on the potential negative effects of fluoride exposure at permissible concentrations (e.g., studies that support water fluoridation), others have shown evidence of fluoride's effects on cellular processes at biologically relevant concentrations. When discussing these controversial results, it is important to highlight that fluoride must be actively considered as a potent toxic compound in the field of toxicology...

"Fluoride can interact with a wide range of cellular processes such as gene expression, cell cycle, proliferation and migration, respiration, metabolism, ion transport, secretion, endocytosis, apoptosis/necrosis, and oxidative stress, and that these mechanisms are involved in a wide variety of signaling pathways."[15]

Fluoride Inhibits the Enzyme Enolase

"Although the toxicity of fluoride is well known, it has been ignored for a long time... As a result, the consumption of fluoride by humans became uncontrolled and unpredictable, often exceeding its therapeutic window," say the authors of the 2012 scientific review, "Molecular Mechanisms of Cytotoxicity and Apoptosis Induced by Inorganic Fluoride." The Russian researchers detail the many ways fluoride harms life. One mechanism: "Fluoride is a well-known inhibitor of enzymes of the glycolytic pathway, first of all enolase."[16]

"Inhibition of glycolysis by fluoride is central to the concept that the anti-microbial effect of fluoride has a role in caries prevention," reported Canada's leading dental journal, *Oral Health*. The bacterium that inhabits the human mouth, *Streptococcus mutans*, causes dental caries by converting dietary sugars into enamel-corroding lactic acid. Fluoride interferes with the complete breakdown of glucose by inhibiting enolase, an intermediary enzyme in the pathway. This results in a reduction in the synthesis of lactic acid and in a significant reduction in the metabolic activity of the cariogenic bacteria.[17]

Fluoride's inhibition of enolase, however, is not limited just to the mouth. Exposure of red blood cells (erythrocytes) to fluoride produces a variety of metabolic alterations.[18]

Via its effect on enolase in human red blood cells, fluoride inhibits active sodium transport, aerobic glucose utilization, and lactate formation.[19,20]

Working with red blood cells of rats, researchers found that sodium fluoride leads to impairment of the cellular antioxidant system; severe energy depletion; and triggers rapid progression of cell death in a dose- and time-dependent manner. Long-term intoxication of the rats with fluoride triggers premature death of their erythrocytes due to intrinsic death-associated biochemical defects and development of anemia.[21-23]

Fluoride, Anemia, and Preterm Birth: A.K. Susheela's Research

Anemia is a condition marked by a deficiency of red blood cells or of hemoglobin, the red protein in blood cells responsible for transporting oxygen in the blood. Anemia is common in pregnancy, because a woman needs to have enough red blood cells to carry oxygen around her body and to her baby.

The leading expert on the connection between fluoride, anemia, and preterm birth is A.K. Susheela, PhD, who has spent more than 25 years researching fluoride toxicity and has over 80 scientific publications in Western and Indian journals. She is executive director of the Fluorosis Research and Rural Development Foundation in India, winner of the 2013 Spirit of Humanity Award in Women's Health presented by AmeriCares India.

"There is now ample scientific evidence to support the fact that ingestion of fluoride prevents biosynthesis of hemoglobin, leading to anemia in human beings," says Susheela.[24] "Fluoride decreases production of erythrocytes (red blood cells) by the bone marrow and other hemopoietic tissues and increases erythrocyte abnormalities resulting in premature death of red blood cells."[25]

In 2010, Susheela conducted a clinical program that emphasized a greatly reduced intake of fluoride and the inclusion of essential nutrients in the daily diet during pregnancy. "Effective Interventional Approach to Control Anemia in Pregnant Women" was the first report dealing with fluoride, pregnancy, anemia, low birthweight babies and the linkages to act upon for the benefit of maternal and reproductive child health programs.[26]

The 205 pregnant women in the study were all anemic. Their hemoglobin levels were less than 9 g/dl, and their urinary fluoride levels were more than 1 mg/l. Ninety pregnant women formed the sample group, and 115 formed the control group. "The major focus of the investigation of the sample group was to eliminate ingestion of fluoride as much as possible," says Susheela. "The sample group was counseled to avoid consumption of fluoride-containing food, water, and other substances." They even changed their toothpaste to a low-fluoride paste. The women were also counseled to ensure an adequate intake of essential nutrients: calcium, vitamins, and antioxidants from dairy products, fruits, and vegetables. The women in the control group were not counseled, but both groups received the standard iron and folic acid tablets.[25,26]

By the time of delivery, improvements in the women's body-mass index were considerably better in the sample group than in the control group, suggesting that the sample group was absorbing nutrients more efficiently. Also, hemoglobin increased by an average of 78% in the sample group compared to 57% in the controls.

> "A striking impact of these interventions for improving the gestation period was also noted." In the sample group, 32% of the women delivered before 37 weeks – compared to 50% in the control group.[25,26]

At the Global Maternal Health Conference convened in New Delhi in 2010, Susheela presented results of a similar but larger study of 481 pregnant women, further confirming:

> "Maternal and child under-nutrition and anemia is not necessarily due to insufficient food intake, but because of the derangement of nutrient absorption due to damage caused to GI mucosa by ingestion of an undesirable chemical substance, namely fluoride through food, water and other sources."[26,27]

Prenatal Fluoride Linked to Low Birthweight
In Susheela's clinical study, the number of low birthweight babies was reduced to 22% in the sample groups of mothers who avoided fluoride, as opposed to 52% in the control groups.[26]

A 2011 study with 108 pregnant women (17-36 years old) concluded: "With increased serum fluoride in the mother, there is an inclination towards preterm delivery, low birthweight, and poor APGAR count."[28] APGAR evaluates a newborn's appearance, pulse, grimace, activity, and respiration.

A 2012 case-control study found a significant association between fluoride levels in the drinking water consumed, dental fluorosis in mothers, and low birthweight of newborns.[29]

Low Birthweight, Cognitive Problems, Autism, and Obesity
Links between low birthweight and a range of motor and cognitive problems have been well known for some time. The 2007 National Summit on America's Children presented an analysis of 35 years of data on more than 12,000 individuals – the first to link birthweight with adult health and socioeconomic success, using a full nationally representative sample of the US population. Some findings:

"Compared to their normal birth weight siblings, low birthweight children are 30 percent less likely to be in excellent or very good health in childhood. They also score significantly lower on reading, passage comprehension, and math achievement tests... Low birthweight children are nearly twice as likely as their normal birth weight siblings to be in problematic health by ages 37-52."[30]

In 2011, researchers at the University of Pennsylvania found that the rate of autism spectrum disorder is highly elevated in children and adults who were born at low birthweight. For 21 years, they followed a regional birth cohort of 1,105 children who weighed less than 2,000 grams (4 pounds, 6 ounces) at birth – finding that 5% of the low birthweight children were diagnosed with autism, compared to 1% of the general population.[31]

Low-birthweight infants also have an increased risk for developing adult obesity.[32] Obesity increases the risk of preterm delivery. A 2013 study of 1.5 million deliveries in Sweden found that women with the highest Body Mass Index also had the highest statistical risk of giving preterm birth. Researchers at Karolinska Institutet say that maternal overweight and obesity have replaced smoking as the most important preventable risk factor for adverse pregnancy outcomes in many countries. In the US, where preterm delivery rates are twice as high as in Sweden, 53% of pregnant women are either overweight or obese compared to 34% of pregnant women in Sweden.[33] (Sweden has prohibited water fluoridation since 1971.)

Iron-Deficiency Anemia
Iron is the main constituent of the hemoglobin molecule, hence a deficiency in iron is a major cause of anemia. About half of all pregnant women don't have enough iron in their body. Pregnant women need about twice as much iron as usual, therefore they have a higher risk of iron-deficiency anemia, which can increase the risk of preterm delivery and low birthweight.

As with most mineral nutrients, iron from digested food is absorbed in the intestinal lining by epithelial cells whose microvilli provide the huge surface area needed to efficiently absorb nutrients. "Fluoride not only decreases production of red blood cells by the bone marrow but also destroys microvilli – the microscopic protrusions lining the intestine," notes Dr. Susheela.[34] "Fluoride diminishes beneficial microbial growth in the gut... resulting in poor absorption of nutrients critical for the biosynthesis of hemoglobin."[25]

In June 2013, Susheela and her team submitted to the Indian Council of Medical Research results of a three-year study to correct anemia in more than 2,500 adolescent school children, ages 10 to 17. When fluoride was withdrawn and nutritious food promoted, the children's anemia was corrected. In contrast, anemia continued in the control group that consumed fluoride, even though they ate a nutritious diet.

Microflora in the GI Tract

The human gut is the natural habitat for a large and dynamic bacterial community. Major functions of the gut microflora include metabolic activities that result in salvage of energy and absorbable nutrients. Colonic microorganisms also play a part in vitamin synthesis and in absorption of calcium, magnesium, and iron.[35]

Lactobacillus acidophilus belongs to a group of bacteria that live in the human small intestine. These beneficial microorganisms aid digestion, help maintain a healthy intestinal tract, and prevent harmful bacteria from congregating there. *L. acidophilus* has been shown to increase iron bioavailability in studies with animals.[36]

When children were fed an iron-fortified probiotic milk beverage supplemented with *L. acidophilus*, they "exhibited higher red blood cell status and a positive correlation between iron intake and hemoglobin" – evidence to support the use of *L. acidophilus* to prevent anemias in children.[37]

When fluoride comes in contact with *L. acidophilus*, it inhibits this beneficial bacterium that aids in the absorption of iron. Fluoride-containing resin-based dental sealants have proved "capable of contact inhibition of *L. acidophilus* and *S. mutans* growth."[38] A statistically significant 49% reduction in *L. acidophilus* counts was obtained 24 hours following mouth rinsing by Egyptian children with 0.05% sodium fluoride solution.[39]

In a 2013 interview, Dr. Susheela explained why India's Iron and Folic Acid Supplementation Program has failed to prevent anemia. As long as fluoride consumption is high, she said:

"No amount of tablets is going to solve anything. Withdrawal of fluoride on the other hand permits the regeneration of microvilli in the gut which improves the absorption of nutrients from the diet and hemoglobin levels improve.

"The evidence is there for the scientific community, bureaucrats, and policymakers, but no one has reproduced it nationally or globally. They're simply not willing to accept the truth."[34]

Thyroid Disorders and Preterm Birth
Subclinical hypothyroidism is associated with an increasing number of adverse effects including infertility, miscarriage, and preterm birth.[40] In a 2005 study of 25,756 women, preterm birth was almost two-fold higher in women with subclinical hypothyroidism compared to women with normal thyroid-stimulating hormone levels.[41]

Each year in the US, at least 80,000 pregnant women have thyroid diseases. A 2013 analysis of 223,512 pregnancies in the United States (2002-2008) found that women with thyroid disorders face greater risk of preterm birth and other complications that have short- and long-term consequences for the health of mother and child, including preeclampsia.[42]

Anemia is often the first sign of hypothyroidism,[43] perhaps in part because thyroid hormones modulate the glycolytic enzyme enolase.[44]

Because of its antagonism to iodine, fluoride has long been known to interfere with the function of the thyroid gland.[45] In 2006, the US National Research Council found substantial evidence that fluoride exposure can impact thyroid function in some individuals. Furthermore, in pregnant women, subclinical hypothyroidism is associated with "decreased IQ of their offspring."[46]

A 2015 study found that high rates of hypothyroidism were at least 30% more likely in areas with water fluoride levels above 0.3 mg/l.[47]

An under-active thyroid gland is also associated with obesity, and obesity increases the risk of preterm delivery.[33]

Prematurity and Infant Mortality
The main cause of the high US infant mortality rate, when compared with Europe, is the very high percentage of preterm births in the United States. After identifying the top 20 leading causes of infant death, the CDC determined that preterm birth is the most frequent cause of infant death in the United States, accounting for 36% of infant deaths in 2007.[48] Prematurity is the #1 cause of death in the first month of life. In 2008, nearly 10,000 babies in the US died from preterm birth-related causes.[49]

Preterm birth doesn't just affect the mortality of infants. A study of 674,820 individuals born in Sweden (who survived to age one) found that "low gestational age at birth was independently associated with increased mortality in early childhood and young adulthood."[50]

The severity of all the problems associated with being born early depends on the degree of prematurity. A 2012 study of 128,000 New York kids found that "each week of increased gestation from 37-41 weeks showed an added benefit in both reading and math scores."[51]

Water Fluoridation and Preterm Birth Rates
A 2009 public-health study, Relationship Between Municipal Water Fluoridation and Preterm Birth in Upstate New York, was undertaken by researchers from the Department of Epidemiology & Biostatistics at the State University of New York (SUNY), because:

> "Current literature suggests an association between periodontal disease and preterm birth. Domestic water fluoridation is thought to have lessened the burden of dental disease. Theoretically, one would expect water fluoridation to be protective against preterm birth."[52]

What was found however surprised the researchers, who did not expect fluoridated water to be positively associated with preterm birth rates – yet they had to conclude otherwise:

> "Domestic water fluoridation was independently associated with an increased risk of preterm birth in logistic regression, after controlling for age, race/ethnicity, neighborhood poverty level, hypertension, and diabetes."[52]

Results of this study were presented at the 2009 American Public Health Association Meeting, but subsequently were never published. One can't help but wonder how much other fluoride research goes unpublished, when results don't support expectations. Case in point:

> The 2007 Oregon Smile Survey showed that non-fluoridated Portland had lower rates of tooth decay. After fluoridation promoters were confronted with this reality check, they omitted Portland statistics from their next survey (2012). When a journalist compared tooth-decay rates of children living in fluoridated vs. nonfluoridated areas of Oregon, fluoridated students averaged a 9% higher decay experience than unfluoridated kids living in the Portland water district (52.03% vs. 47.81%).[53]

After the SUNY public health study, a logical next step would have been to look at available data for ecological associations elsewhere in the US. According to CDC data for 2010, in the 25 least fluoridated states (average fluoridation rate: 52%), the preterm birth rate averaged 116 per 1,000 births. In the 25 most fluoridated states (average fluoridation rate: 90%), the preterm birth rate averaged 5% higher: 122 per 1,000 births.[54,55]

If that difference of six births per 1,000 were extrapolated to the United States, where four million births occurred in 2010 (when 66% of the population was fluoridated), then higher levels of water fluoridation would be associated that year with about 16,000 more preterm births – each one with an annual societal economic burden of more than $50,000.[2]

Although this nationwide statistical association is not adjusted for age, race, poverty, and maternal disease (as the SUNY study was), nevertheless it is the best large-scale population data we have – a snapshot that supports laboratory and clinical studies showing an association between fluoridated water and preterm birth. It should not be dismissed, but after the SUNY study, no further research has been published.

Similar statistical snapshots of America in 2010 reveal that low-birthweight rates averaged 5% higher, and infant mortality rates averaged 17% higher in the 25 most-fluoridated states compared to the 25 least-fluoridated states. Neonatal (under 28 days) deaths were 19% higher.[56,57]

Fluoridated water's multiple correlations with *life decay* make a far more compelling case to halt fluoridation, than its single correlation with tooth decay did to start fluoridation in 1945. (See pages 74-76).

Link Between Preterm Birth and Brain Disorders
In 2012, researchers at the University of Adelaide discovered a possible mechanistic link between the altered brain physiology of preterm birth and subsequent neurological deficits. Their research provides the first physiological evidence that human adolescents who were born preterm have a "significantly reduced capacity for cortical neuroplasticity." Dr. Julia Pitcher of the Robinson Institute says plasticity in the brain is vital for learning and memory throughout life. "It enables the brain to reorganize itself, responding to changes in environment, behavior and stimuli by modifying the number and strength of connections between neurons and different brain areas."[58]

"The growth of the brain is rapid between 20 and 37 weeks gestation, Pitcher said. "Being born even mildly preterm appears to subtly but significantly alter brain microstructure, neural connectivity, and neurochemistry." In contrast, the brains of term-born teenagers were highly plastic.[58]

This study's findings also suggested a mechanism. Altered hypothalamic-pituitary-adrenal (HPA) axis function due to preterm birth may be "a significant modulator of this altered neuroplasticity." The HPA axis a complex neurohormone mechanism that regulates metabolic and behavioral reactions to physiological and environmental stress. It is highly susceptible to programming during fetal and neonatal development.

Animal and human studies have demonstrated that stress associated with preterm birth provokes adaptive changes in endocrine and metabolic processes that become permanently programmed via the HPA axis – affecting later health, memory, learning, executive function, and associated behavior throughout life.[59-61]

Premature birth is a stressful event, not only due to a shortened gestation period, but also because of medical interventions during the first weeks of life (painful procedures, handling, mechanical ventilation, maternal separation).

Abnormal regulation of the HPA axis is commonly associated with a range of affective and stress-related disorders. A 2012 Swedish study of more than a million individuals found that preterm birth was significantly associated with increased risk of psychiatric hospitalization in adulthood across a range of psychiatric disorders.[62]

HPA Axis and the Gut
"The gut microbiota contributes to developmental programming; a process whereby an environmental factor acting during a developmental 'window of vulnerability' can have a potentially life-long impact on physiological function," say researchers at the Brain-Body Institute at McMaster University in Ontario, Canada. The presence of gut microbiota regulates the set point for HPA axis activity.[63,64] (See also pages 51-52.)

Findings from a 2004 study "suggest that exposure to indigenous microbiota at an early developmental stage, when brain plasticity may still be preserved, is required for the HPA system to become fully susceptible to inhibitory neural regulation."[65]

Attention-Deficit Hyperactivity Disorder (ADHD)

In a study of boys with ADHD and disruptive behavior symptoms, those scoring high on "callous unemotional traits" showed a blunted HPA axis reactivity to the experimentally induced stress.[66]

In the US, ADHD is the most common neurodevelopmental disorder of childhood, affecting about 7% of all children. In 2013, the results of a long-running study (5,718 children in Rochester, Minnesota born from 1976 through 1982) found that 29% of the children with ADHD still had ADHD as adults. Of the children who still had ADHD as adults, 81% had at least one other psychiatric disorder, as compared with 47% of those who no longer had ADHD and 35% of controls. Lead investigator, William Barbaresi, MD, says, "We suffer from the misconception that ADHD is just an annoying childhood disorder that's overtreated. This couldn't be further from the truth."[67]

Premature infants have significantly more severe symptoms of ADHD at school age.[68] Another statistical snapshot of America reveals that children's ADHD rates[69] averaged about 14% higher in the 25 most-fluoridated states compared to the 25 least-fluoridated states.

A 2015 study found that for each one-percent increase in artificial fluoridation prevalence in 1992 was associated with approximately 67,000 to 131,000 additional ADHD diagnoses (2003 to 2011).[70]

Prenatal Fluoride and Hyperactivity

A landmark study led by Phyllis Mullenix, PhD, found that rats exposed prenatally to fluoride exhibit higher levels of hyperactivity.[71] After her research was published in *Neurotoxicology and Teratology* (1995), Mullenix was fired from Boston's Forsyth Dental Center, where for 10 years she had been Head of the Toxicology Department. As documented by investigative journalist Christopher Bryson in *The Fluoride Deception*, Forsyth's associate director told Mullenix:

> "You are going against what the dentists and everybody have been publishing for fifty years, that this is safe and effective. You must be wrong. You are jeopardizing the financial support of this entire institution. If you publish these studies, NIDR [National Institute of Dental Research] is not going to fund anymore research at Forsyth." (Forsyth was getting about 90% of its money from NIDR.)[72]

By 2010, more than 80 animal studies had confirmed what Mullenix et al. reported.[73] Also, the Neurotoxicology Division of the EPA had found "substantial evidence" that fluoride is a chemical "toxic to the developing mammalian nervous system." (See pages 3, 53-54.)

Note: rat studies involving higher doses of fluoride are relevant to humans, because research shows that when rats consumed 75-125 ppm and humans 5-10 ppm fluoride in their respective drinking waters, the result was equivalent ranges of plasma fluoride levels.[74]

Fluoride, Defective Tooth Enamel, and Prematurity
A major 2011 European review of fluoride's health effects concluded: "Systemic exposure to fluoride through drinking water is associated with an increased risk of dental and bone fluorosis in a dose-response manner without a detectable threshold."[75]

Studies show that the prevalence and severity of developmental defects of enamel (DDE) in children increase significantly with the increase in fluoride levels in drinking water, as well as with the ingestion of fluoride tablets.[76-78]

Premature infants are more frequently affected by tooth enamel anomalies or defects when compared with infants born at term. An Australian study of 8,411 children found the prevalence of DDE in children and adolescents born prematurely was 56.5%, while the control group was 9.3%.[79] (See also pages 56-57.)

Low-birthweight children more likely than their normal birthweight counterparts to have enamel hypoplasia, a form of DDE in which the tooth enamel is hard but thin and deficient in amount.[80]

Developmental enamel defects in primary teeth have been found at least twice as frequently in children with mental retardation.[81] Another statistical snapshot of America reveals that children's mental retardation rates in 1993 averaged 33% higher in the 26 states fluoridated above the average national level, compared to the 24 least-fluoridated states. Twenty years later it averaged 57% higher![82]

Genetic Factors
Animal studies show there is a genetic component in the pathogenesis of dental fluorosis and in bone response to fluoride exposure. Different strains of inbred mice demonstrate differential physiological responses to ingested fluoride.[83,84]

In human populations, African Americans appear to be more vulnerable to fluoride's toxicity. They have higher rates of dental fluorosis as well as preterm birth. A study of 83 African American and 109 White children (7-14 years old) found that even though both groups had the same water and saliva fluoride concentrations, dental fluorosis was observed in 63% of White children, but in 80% of African American children.[85]

"Approximately 50% of preterm birth has no clear medical cause, and evidence strongly suggests that genetic factors contribute to some of these cases," says Dartmouth Professor of Genetics Scott Williams, PhD. It's unknown why preterm birth happens in about 10% of pregnancies in Caucasian women nationwide, but in about 20% of pregnancies of African-American women.[86]

When a genetic predisposition is combined with mild inflammation, the rate of preterm birth profoundly increases in mice. Researchers observed aspects of the same molecular signatures in tissue samples of women who had undergone preterm birth: increases in cyclooxygenase-2 (COX-2) signaling.[87] Fluorides have well-established ability to cause and aggravate inflammation,[15] including increased expression of COX-2 in human cells.[88]

We really don't know the racial and genetic factors that determine an individual's resistance to developing fluorosis and susceptibility to fluoride's multiple mechanisms of toxicity in the body and brain.[15,16]

Fluoride Contaminates US Processed Food and Beverage Chain
Americans consume uncontrolled and unknown amounts of fluoride. Water is the predominant source of fluoride in the United States, however, a historically unprecedented array of other sources are responsible for a significant exposure to fluoride, especially in processed foods and beverages.

> In 2006, the National Research Council said manufacturers should provide information on the fluoride content of commercial foods and beverages. (See Appendix B.) A decade later, fluoride content is still missing from food ingredient labels, including pet foods whose very high fluoride content has been implicated in canine bone cancer.[89,90]

Other sources of fluoride exposure include toothpaste, mouthwash, supplements, and other dental products and treatments; fluorinated pharmaceuticals, pesticides, and post-harvest fumigants. The additive effect can be substantial.

In 1993, the National Research Council admitted, "It is no longer feasible to estimate with reasonable accuracy the level of fluoride exposure simply on the basis of concentration in drinking water supply."[91] Therefore, even where fluoride levels in drinking water are claimed to be safe, mothers-to-be should take steps to minimize their consumption of fluoride to reduce the risk of premature birth – especially if they have dental fluorosis, visible proof of one's susceptibility to systemic fluoride toxicity.

Residence in the US is a risk factor for preterm birth, and more people consume artificially fluoridated water (and products made with it) in America alone than in the rest of the world combined.[92] It is high time we change our long habit of not thinking fluoride consumption wrong and realize it is a significant risk factor for premature birth and long-term neurological disabilities.

A vibrant fully functioning brain is the most precious gift of life. It is inexcusable to promote, condone, or ignore any substance or policy that threatens this birthright.

* * * * *

Correlations Between
Cognitive Scores and Gestational Age

A major study published in 2002 in the
Journal of the American Medical Association:

"We report the first meta-analysis on the cognitive and behavioral outcomes of school-aged children who were born preterm by combining the results from case-control studies published between 1980 and November 2001...

"Among 1556 cases and 1720 controls, controls had significantly higher cognitive scores compared with children who were born preterm...

"Conclusions: Children who were born preterm are at risk for reduced cognitive test scores and their immaturity at birth is directly proportional to the mean cognitive scores at school age. Preterm-born children also show an increased incidence of ADHD and other behaviors."[93]

References – Fluoride, Premature Birth and Impaired Neurodevelopment

1. Institute of Medicine (US) Committee on Understanding Premature Birth and Assuring Healthy Outcomes; Behrman RE, Butler AS, editors. Preterm Birth: Causes, Consequences, and Prevention. Washington (DC): National Academies Press (US); 2007. Appendix B, Chapters 11 and 12.

2. Patoine B. The vulnerable premature brain: Rapid neural development in third trimester heightens brain risks. Dana Foundation. May 2010.

3. Slegers M. Imaging technique shows premature birth interrupts vital brain development processes leading to reduced cognitive abilities in infants. King's College London press release. May 20, 2013.

4. Ball G, Srinivasan L, Aljabar P, et al. Development of cortical microstructure in the preterm human brain. *Proc Natl Acad Sci USA*. 2013 June 4;110(23):9541–9546.

5. Born too soon: The global action report of preterm birth. World Health Organization. May 2, 2012.

6. McNeil DG. U.S. lags in global measure of premature births. *New York Times*. May 2, 2012.

7. Lynch E. New global report says US lags behind 130 other nations in preterm birth rate. March of Dimes Foundation press release. May 2, 2012.

8. Bendure V. Study finds residence in US a risk factor for preterm birth. Society for Maternal-Fetal Medicine press release. February 9, 2012.

9. Chang HH, Larson J, Blencowe H, et al. Preventing preterm births: Analysis of trends and potential reductions with interventions in 39 countries with very high human development index. *Lancet.* 2013 Jan 19;381(9862): 223–234.

10. Lawn J. Best-available science will allow just 5 percent relative reduction in high-income countries' preterm birth rates by 2015. *The Lancet* press release. November 15, 2012.

11. Breaker RR. First person: How we discovered fluoride riboswitches. Yale News. December 22, 2011.

12. Breaker RR. New insight on the response of bacteria to fluoride. *Caries Res*. 2012;46(1):78–81.

13. Keeley J. Bacteria battle against toxic fluoride. Howard Hughes Medical Institute press release. December 22, 2011.

14. Kresge N. Fighting fluoride: Riboswitch helps bacteria toss out toxic fluoride. Howard Hughes Medical Institute Bulletin. May 2012. Vol. 25/#2.

15. Barbier O, Arreola-Mendoza L, Del Razo LM. Molecular mechanisms of fluoride toxicity. *Chemico-Biological Inter*. 2010 Nov 5;188(2):319–333.

16. Agalakova NI, Gusev GP. Molecular mechanisms of cytotoxicity and apoptosis induced by inorganic fluoride. *ISRN Cell Biol*. 2012:403835.

17. Nouri MR, Titley KC. Pediatrics: A review of the antibacterial effect of fluoride. *Oral Health Journal*. January 1, 2003.

18. Feig SA, Shohet SB, Nathan DG. Energy metabolism in human erythrocytes. I. Effects of sodium fluoride. *J Clin Invest*. 1971 Aug;50(8): 1731–1737.

19. Millman MS, Omachi A. The role of oxidized nicotinamide adenine dinucleotide in fluoride inhibition of active sodium transport in human erythrocytes. *J Gen Physiol*. 1972 Sep;60(3):337–350.

20. Gumińska M, Sterkowicz J. Effect of sodium fluoride on glycolysis in human erythrocytes and Ehrlich ascites tumour cells in vitro. *Acta Biochim Pol*. 1976;23(4):285–291.

21. Agalakova NI, Gusev GP. Fluoride induces oxidative stress and ATP depletion in the rat erythrocytes in vitro. *Environ Toxicol Pharmacol*. 2012 Sep;34(2):334–337.

22. Agalakova NI, Gusev GP. Fluoride-induced death of rat erythrocytes in vitro. *Toxicol In Vitro*. 2011 Dec;25(8):1609–1618.

23. Agalakova NI, Gusev GP. Excessive fluoride consumption leads to accelerated death of erythrocytes and anemia in rats. *Biol Trace Elem Res*. 2013 Jun;153(1-3):340–349.

24. Page A. Fluorosis: Crippling the innocent. *Asian Geographic Magazine*. 2010;73(4):112–117. Reports and interviews given by Prof. A.K. Susheela to the media.

25. Susheela AK. Anemia in pregnancy: An easily rectifiable problem (Guest editorial). *Fluoride* April-June 2010 43(2)104–107.

26. Susheela AK, Mondal NK, Gupta R, et al. Effective interventional approach to control anaemia in pregnant women. *Current Science*. 25 May 2010;98(10).

27. A. Susheela: A novel and effective interventional approach for prevention and control of anemia in pregnancy and low birth weight babies. Presentations: The importance of maternal nutrition for maternal health. August 31, 2010. Global Maternal Health Conference. New Delhi, India.

28. Gurumurthy SM, Mohanty S, Bhongir AV, Mishra AK, Rao P. Association of higher maternal serum fluoride with adverse fetal outcomes. *Int. J. Med. Public Health*. April-June 2011: Vol 1; Issue 2.

29. Diouf M, Cisse D, Lo CM, Ly M, Faye D, Ndiaye O. Pregnant women living in areas of endemic fluorosis in Senegal and low birthweight newborns: Case-control study. *Rev Epidemiol Sante Publique*. 2012 Apr; 60(2):103–108.

30. Swanbrow D. Born to lose: How birth weight affects adult health and success. University of Michigan News. June 5, 2007.

31. Pinto-Martin JA, Levy SE, Feldman JF, et al. Prevalence of autism spectrum disorder in adolescents born weighing <2000 grams. *Pediatrics*. 2011 Nov;128(5):883–891.

32. Mecoy L. LA Biomed study increases understanding of link between low birth weights and obesity later in life. LA Biomedical Research Institute press release. June 21, 2011.

 Desai M, Li T, Ross MG. Hypothalamic neurosphere progenitor cells in low birth-weight rat newborns: neurotrophic effects of leptin and insulin. Brain Res. 2011 Mar 10;1378:29–42.

33. Obesity increases the risk of preterm delivery. Karolinska Institutet press release. June 11, 2013.

 Cnattingius S. Maternal overweight and obesity during pregnancy associated with increased risk of preterm delivery. The *JAMA* Network Journals press release. June 11, 2013.

34. Dutta N. Why the Govt's Iron and Folic Acid Supplementation Programme won't produce desired results (Exclusive interview with Dr A.K. Susheela). HealthSite.com. August 6, 2013.

 Video interview with A.K. Susheela. "Today Tonight" from Australia's Adelaide 7 television news program. July 22, 2010.

35. Guarner F, Malagelada JR. Gut flora in health and disease. *Lancet*. 2003 Feb 8;361(9356):512–519.

36. Oda T, Kado-oka Y, Hashiba H. Effect of Lactobacillus acidophilus on iron bioavailability in rats. *J Nutr Sci Vitaminol (Tokyo)*. 1994 Dec;40(6): 613–616.

37. Silva MR, Dias G, Ferreira CL, Franceschini SC, Costa NM. Growth of preschool children was improved when fed an iron-fortified fermented milk beverage supplemented with Lactobacillus acidophilus. *Nutr Res*. 2008 Apr; 28(4):226–232.

Mitchell, J. Prebiotics and probiotics in young children. *Natural Medicine Journal*. October 2010. Vol. 2 Issue 10.

38. Naorungroj S, Wei HH, Arnold RR, Swift EJ Jr, Walter R. Antibacterial surface properties of fluoride-containing resin-based sealants. *J Dent.* 2010 May;38(5):387–391.

39. Waly NG. Assessment of salivary Lactobacillus and Streptococcus mutans counts following sodium fluoride mouthrinsing in Egyptian children. *Egypt Dent J.* 1995 Apr;41(2):1179–1188.

40. Milanesi A, Brent GA. Management of hypothyroidism in pregnancy. *Curr Opin Endocrinol Diabetes Obes.* 2011 Oct;18(5):304–309.

41. Casey BM, Dashe JS, Wells CE, et al. Subclinical hypothyroidism and pregnancy outcomes. *Obstet Gynecol.* 2005 Feb;105(2):239–245.

42. Gingery JG. Thyroid conditions raise risk of pregnancy complications: Hormone disorders linked to higher rates of preterm birth, preeclampsia. The Endocrine Society press release. May 29, 2013.

   Männistö T, Mendola P, Grewal J, Xie Y, Chen Z, Laughon SK. Thyroid diseases and adverse pregnancy outcomes in a contemporary US cohort. *J Clin Endocrinol Metab.* 2013 Jul;98(7):2725–2733.

   See also: Korevaar TI, Schalekamp-Timmermans S, de Rijke YB, et al. Hypothyroxinemia and TPO-antibody positivity are risk factors for premature delivery: The Generation R study. *J Clin Endocrinol Metab.* 2013 Nov;98(11):4382–4390.

43. Erdogan M, Aybike K, Ganıdagli S, Mustafa K. Characteristics of anemia in subclinical and overt hypothyroid patients. *Endocr J.* 2012;59(3):213-220.

44. Merkulova T, Keller A, Oliviero P, et al. Thyroid hormones differentially modulate enolase isozymes during rat skeletal and cardiac muscle development. *Am J Physiol Endocrinol Metab.* 2000 Feb;278(2):E330–339.

45. Schuld A. History of the fluoride/iodine antagonism. Parents of Fluoride Poisoned Children. 2013.

46. National Research Council. *Fluoride in drinking water: A scientific review of EPA's standards.* Effects of thyroid function. National Academies Press;2006:236.

47. Water fluoridation in England linked to higher rates of underactive thyroid: switch to other approaches in bid to protect tooth health, say researchers. *British Medical Journal* press release. February 23, 2015.

Peckham S, Lowery D, Spencer S. Are fluoride levels in drinking water associated with hypothyroidism prevalence in England? A large observational study of GP practice data and fluoride levels in drinking water. *J Epidemiol Community Health* 2015;0:1–6.

48. Behind international rankings of infant mortality: How the United States compares with Europe. National Center for Health Statistics. Nov. 2009.

Callaghan WM, MacDorman MF, Rasmussen SA, Qin C, Lackritz EM. The contribution of preterm birth to infant mortality rates in the United States. *Pediatrics.* 2006 Oct;118(4):1566–1573.

49. Preventing Preterm Births Saves Babies' Lives. March of Dimes. September 4, 2012.

50. Crump C, Sundquist K, Sundquist J, Winkleby MA. Gestational age at birth and mortality in young adulthood. *JAMA.* 2011;306(11):1233–1240.

51. Noble KG, Fifer WP, Rauh VA, Nomura Y, Andrews HF. Academic achievement varies with gestational age among children born at term. *Pediatrics.* 2012 Aug;130(2):e257–264.

Boyle C. Smart babies stay in the womb longer. *New York Daily News.* July 2, 2012.

52. Hart R, Feelemyer J, Gray C, et al. Relationship between municipal water fluoridation and preterm birth in Upstate New York, 2009. American Public Health Association Meeting and Expo. No.9, 2009.

53. Bailey-Shah S. Before you vote: Fluoride and kids' teeth – what does the data show? *KATU News.* Portland, Oregon. April 25, 2013. (*Cascadia Times*)

54. 2010 Water Fluoridation Statistics. CDC. May 11, 2011.

55. Martin JA, Hamilton BE, Ventura SJ, et al. Births: Final Data for 2010. *Natl Vital Stat Rep.* August 28, 2012;61(01)12, Table E.

56. Kids Count. 2013 Data Book: State Trends in Child Well-Being. Annie E. Casey Foundation. Low birthweight babies. 2010. Page 44.

57. Murphy SL, Xu J, Kochanek KD. Deaths: Final Data for 2010. *Natl Vital Stat Rep.* May 8, 2013;61(04)97, Table 22.

58. Pitcher JB, Riley AM, Doeltgen SH, et al. Physiological evidence consistent with reduced neuroplasticity in human adolescents born preterm. *J Neurosci.* 2012 Nov 14;32(46):16410–16416.

Pitcher JB. Teenagers' brains affected by preterm birth: Why being preterm could impair memory, learning. University of Adelaide press release. November 13, 2012.

59. Phillips DI, Jones A. Fetal programming of autonomic and HPA function: Do people who were small babies have enhanced stress responses? *J Physiol.* 2006 April 1;572(Pt 1):45–50.

60. Sullivan MC, Hawes K, Winchester SB, Miller RJ. Developmental origins theory from prematurity to adult disease. *J Obstet Gynecol Neonatal Nurs.* 2008 Mar–Apr;37(2):158–164.

61. Huang LT. The link between perinatal glucocorticoids exposure and psychiatric disorders. *Pediatric Research* (2011) 69, 19R–25R.

62. Nosarti C, Reichenberg A, Murray RM, et al. Preterm birth and psychiatric disorders in young adult life. *Arch Gen Psychiatry.* 2012;69(6): 610–617.

63. Kunze WA, Forsythe P. Voices from within: Gut microbes and the CNS. *Cell Mol Life Sci.* 2013 Jan;70(1):55–69.

64. Neufeld KM, Kang N, Bienenstock J, Foster JA. Reduced anxiety-like behavior and central neurochemical change in germ-free mice. *Neurogastroenterology & Motility.* Mar 2011;23(3):255–e119.

   Foster JA, Neufeld KM. Gut-brain axis: how the microbiome influences anxiety and depression. *Trends Neurosci.* 2013 May;36(5):305–312.

65. Sudo N, Chida Y, Aiba Y, et al. Postnatal microbial colonization programs the hypothalamic-pituitary-adrenal system for stress response in mice. *J Physiol.* 2004 Jul 1;558(Pt 1):263–275.

66. Stadler C, Kroeger A, Weyers P, et al. Cortisol reactivity in boys with attention-deficit/hyperactivity disorder and disruptive behavior problems: The impact of callous unemotional traits. *Psychiatry Res.* 2011 May 15;187 (1-2):204–209.

67. Weber M. ADHD takes a toll well into adulthood. Boston Children's Hospital press release. March 4, 2013.

68. Chu SM, Tsai MH, Hwang FM, et al. The relationship between attention deficit hyperactivity disorder and premature infants in Taiwanese: A case control study. *BMC Psychiatry.* 2012;12:85.

69. Increasing prevalence of parent-reported attention-deficit/hyperactivity disorder among children – United States, 2003 and 2007. Percent of Youth 4-17 ever diagnosed with attention-deficit/hyperactivity disorder. *Morbidity and Mortality Weekly Report (MMWR).* November 12, 2010;59 (44):1439–1443. Table 3 (2007).

70. Malin AJ, Till C. Exposure to fluoridated water and attention deficit hyperactivity disorder prevalence among children and adolescents in the United States: an ecological association. *Environmental Health* 2015;14:17.

71. Mullenix PJ, Denbesten PK, Schunior A, Kernan WJ. Neurotoxicity of sodium fluoride in rats. *Neurotoxicol Teratol*. 1995 Mar–Apr;17(2):169–177. Full study: www.fluoridealert.org/wp-content/uploads/mullenix-1995.pdf

Fluoride and the Brain: An Interview with Dr. Phyllis Mullenix. Fluoride Action Network. October 18, 1997.

72. Bryson C. *The Fluoride Deception*. Seven Stories Press;2004:22.

73. Connett P, Beck J, Micklem HS. *The case against fluoride: How hazardous waste ended up in our drinking water and the bad science and powerful politics that keep it there*. Chelsea Green Publishing;2010:148–150.

74. Mullenix PJ. Central nervous system damage from fluorides: The neurotoxicity of fluoride. Fluoridation.com. September 14, 1998.

75. Critical review of any new evidence on the hazard profile, health effects, and human exposure to fluoride and the fluoridating agents of drinking water. European Union's Scientific Committee on Health and Environmental Risks (SCHER). 16 May 2011. Abstract.

76. Ekanayake L, van der Hoek W. Dental caries and developmental defects of enamel in relation to fluoride levels in drinking water in an arid area of Sri Lanka. *Caries Res*. 2002 Nov-Dec;36(6):398–404.

77. Wong HM, McGrath C, Lo EC, King NM. Association between developmental defects of enamel and different concentrations of fluoride in the public water supply. *Caries Res*. 2006;40(6):481–486.

78. Hiller KA, Wilfart G, Schmalz G. Developmental enamel defects in children with different fluoride supplementation – a follow-up study. *Caries Res*. 1998;32(6):405–411.

79. Hall RK. Prevalence of developmental defects of tooth enamel (DDE) in a pediatric hospital department of dentistry population (1). *Adv Dent Res*. 1989 Sep;3(2):114–119.

80. Masumo R, Bårdsen A, Astrøm AN. Developmental defects of enamel in primary teeth and association with early life course events: a study of 6–36 month old children in Manyara, Tanzania. *BMC Oral Health*. 2013;13:21.

81. Bhat M, Nelson KB. Developmental enamel defects in primary teeth in children with cerebral palsy, mental retardation, or hearing defects: a review. *Adv Dent Res*. 1989 Sep;3(2):132–142.

82. State-Specific Rates of Mental Retardation – United States, 1993. CDC. *Morbidity and Mortality Weekly Report (MMWR)*. January 26, 1996;45(03):61–65. Table 1: Prevalence rate of mental retardation, by state for children (6–17 years old) per 1,000 population, 1993.

Osmunson B. Comment and advisory: EPA. March 13, 2011. Likely and possible harm to the brain and IQ from fluoride:60. Effect of fluoride on the brain: estimating IQ drop:176–179.

MacArthur JD. Fluoridated Water's Association with Mental Retardation and Intellectual Disability. 2018. PregnancyAndFluorideDoNotMix.com/mentalretardation.html

83. Everett ET. Fluoride's effects on the formation of teeth and bones, and the influence of genetics. *J Dent Res*. 2011 May;90(5):552–560.

Everett ET, McHenry MA, Reynolds N, et al. Dental fluorosis: variability among different inbred mouse strains. *J Dent Res*. 2002 Nov;81(11):794–798.

84. Mousny M, Banse X, Wise L, Everett ET, et al. The genetic influence on bone susceptibility to fluoride. *Bone*. 2006 Dec;39(6):1283–1289.

85. Martinez-Mier EA, Soto-Rojas AE. Differences in exposure and biological markers of fluoride among White and African American children. *J Public Health Dent*. 2010 Summer;70(3):234–240.

86. Hertel D. Dartmouth researchers aim to discover the unknown causes of premature birth. Geisel School of Medicine press release. July 18, 2013.

87. Miller N. Scientists prevent preterm birth caused by gene-environment interactions. Cincinnati Children's Hospital Medical Center press release. August 27, 2013.

88. Ridley W, Matsuoka M. Fluoride-induced cyclooxygenase-2 expression and prostaglandin E2 production in A549 human pulmonary epithelial cells. *Toxicol Lett*. 2009 Aug 10;188(3):180–185.

89. Dog food comparison shows high fluoride levels. Environmental Working Group. June 26, 2009.

90. Glasser G. Dogs, cats, osteosarcoma, dysplasia and pet food fluoride. National Pure Water Association.

91. Committee on Toxicology. Health Effects of Ingested Fluoride. Washington DC: *National Academy Press*;1993:128.

92. Countries that fluoridate their water. Fluoride Action Network. August 2012.

93. Bhutta AT, Cleves MA, Casey PH, Cradock MM, Anand KJ. Cognitive and behavioral outcomes of school-aged children who were born preterm: a meta-analysis. *JAMA*. 2002 Aug 14; 288(6):728–737.

Chapter 2

New research and diverse evidence implicate fluoride and fluorosis in the pathogenesis of preeclampsia, the dangerous pregnancy complication caused by the abnormal placenta.

An earlier version of this report was
published in the May 2015 *Townsend Letter:
The Examiner of Alternative Medicine*

Placental Fluorosis: Fluoride and Preeclampsia

Eclampsia, a convulsive disorder of pregnancy, was described by ancient civilizations of China, Egypt, and India. Late in the 19th century, it was recognized that eclampsia was preceded by new onset hypertension during the second half of pregnancy, hence the term *preeclampsia*.[1] Preeclampsia is associated with high maternal and fetal/neonatal morbidity and mortality, especially in developing countries.

Each year in the United States, preeclampsia is responsible for approximately 18% of all maternal deaths and more than 10,000 infant deaths. Increasing since 1980, preeclampsia and related hypertensive disorders of pregnancy impact about 5-8% of all births in the US, whose infant mortality rate is one of the highest in the industrialized world.[2]

The root cause of this life-threatening pregnancy complication is the abnormal placenta. Its removal puts an end to the disease. Despite a long history and extensive research, the true pathogenesis of preeclampsia remains unknown.

Something else that has been around for millennia is fluoride and fluorosis, the visible evidence of an individual's susceptibility to fluoride's adverse systemic effects, but they have never been associated with preeclampsia... nor ruled out... nor even considered – although US fluoride researchers have long known that the placentas of women who drink fluoridated water contain significantly higher concentrations of fluoride.

In a 1952 issue of *Science* magazine, Harold C. Hodge (chief toxicologist for the US Army's Manhattan Project) reported that women who drank water artificially fluoridated with 1.0-1.2 mg/l (milligram per liter) of fluoride averaged 2 ppm (parts per million) fluoride in their placentas, compared with 0.74 ppm fluoride in the placentas of women who drank nonfluoridated water. Maternal blood fluoride levels were also nearly three times higher because of fluoridated water (0.040 vs. 0.014 ppm).[3]

More recent clinical research shows that the placenta can accumulate fluoride in healthy women who are exposed in pregnancy to relatively low fluoride concentrations in water and in air. The placenta acts as a natural barrier to the passage of larger quantities of fluoride to the fetus. Fluoride content of the placenta can be significantly higher than that of maternal serum.[4]

Preeclampsia is a progressive disorder with mild to severe consequences, and epidemiological studies clearly confirm that genetic factors are involved.[5] Dental fluorosis also has mild to severe consequences, and animal studies show that there is a genetic component in the pathogenesis of dental fluorosis and in bone response to fluoride exposure.[6]

In humans, "severity of dental fluorosis varies individually at the same level of intake."[7] Black children in the US have significantly higher rates and more severe forms of dental fluorosis than either white or Hispanic children, and it is not known why.[8]

Compared to other races, African American women in the US have higher rates of preeclampsia, and its effects present earlier and are more severe. Their death rate from preeclampsia is three times higher, and it is not known why.[9,10]

Most fluoride research is dental research, especially in countries that artificially fluoridate their drinking water. During the first 7 months of 2018, PubMed shows 1,540 studies were published that have *placenta* in their title or abstract. For *fluoride*: 1,145. For *placenta* AND *fluoride*: just a single study was published (and only 4 in the previous decade). One was relevant to preeclampsia: Tskitishvili et al., 2010. (See page 36.)

Very little is known about how the human placenta is affected by fluoride's multiple mechanisms of cytotoxicity,[11] but placental fluorosis is certainly a possibility. Like dental fluorosis, a woman's vulnerability to placental fluorosis would depend on individual genetic, metabolic, and environmental factors.

ER Stress – Link Between Fluorosis and Preeclampsia
This century's science is revealing that preeclampsia and dental fluorosis share the same key subcellular mechanism of pathophysiology: endoplasmic reticulum stress. Within a cell, the endoplasmic reticulum (ER) is the organelle responsible for the biosynthesis, folding, and assembly of all secretory and membrane-bound proteins. ER function is highly sensitive to extracellular stimuli. During environmental, developmental, or genetic stress, the cell's folding capacity can become overwhelmed and cause misfolded proteins to accumulate, a condition known as ER stress.[12,13]

Buhimschi et al. (2014) identified misfolded proteins specific to preeclampsia in the urine of pregnant women weeks before their preeclampsia becomes clinically apparent.[14] Note: early in the 20th century, proteinuria (abnormal quantities of protein in the urine) was identified as a cardinal feature of preeclampsia.[1]

ER stress activates a defense mechanism called the "unfolded protein response" that reduces protein synthesis to decrease the burden on the ER. Cells with high secretory activity have a large amount of ER and are more susceptible to ER stress. These include ameloblasts, osteoblasts, and trophoblasts.

Fluoride Causes ER Stress in Dental and Skeletal Fluorosis
Ameloblasts are cells present during tooth development that secrete large amounts of proteins that later mineralize to form tooth enamel.

Researchers at the Forsyth Institute in Massachusetts, a fluoride research center for the past century, found that fluoride initiates an ER stress response in ameloblasts that interferes with protein synthesis and secretion – culminating in dental fluorosis. Beginning with the lowest dose tested, they observed an increase in the magnitude of ER stress with increasing doses of fluoride.[15]

Osteoblasts are cells that secrete the protein matrix for bone formation. In its comprehensive 2006 report, "Fluoride in Drinking Water," the US National Research Council (NRC) said, "Fluoride is a biologically active ion with demonstrable effects on bone cells, both osteoblasts and osteoclasts."[16] In the pathogenesis of skeletal fluorosis, fluoride causes ER stress during osteoblast maturation.[17]

The area enclosed by the membrane of the ER includes a network of interconnecting flattened sac-like structures called *cisternae*. Fluoride has been shown to cause dilated cisternae in the brains of rats, as well as in the brain tissue of human fetuses from an endemic fluorosis area.[18,19] In fetuses whose mothers had dental fluorosis, the major subcellular pathology was varying degrees of cistern dilation in epithelial cells of livers, adrenal glands, and thyroid glands.[20]

ER Stress in Preeclampsia
Trophoblasts are the precursor cells of the human placenta. The extensive secretory activity of syncytiotrophoblasts, the outer trophoblast layer responsible for nutrient exchange, renders them vulnerable to ER stress.

> ER stress is specific to syncytiotrophoblasts, the cells in direct contact with maternal blood, the source of fluoride exposure.[20b]

At the University of Cambridge's Center for Trophoblast Research, Burton and Yung confirmed high levels of ER stress in placentas from cases of early-onset preeclampsia (<34 weeks of gestation). Reduced protein synthesis caused by ER stress has a severe detrimental effect on placental development by causing decreased levels of many hormones, growth factors, and regulatory proteins – all of which lead to the placental insufficiency and dysfunction in preeclampsia.[21]

Electron micrographs of syncytiotrophoblasts in the normal placenta show the cisternae have only minimal dilation. In preeclamptic placentas, however, the cisternae are widely dilated.[21]

Fluoride: Hypertension, Arterial Stiffness, and Preeclampsia
The primary pathological feature of preeclampsia is hypertension. Many studies have found a positive correlation between increased prevalence of hypertension with increased concentrations of fluoride in drinking water, as well as with fluorosis in the human body.[22]

The risk of hypertension prevalence increased by 25% when fluoride levels in drinking water increased from 0.84 to 1.55 mg/l.[23] Note: for many decades, US drinking water was 'optimally' fluoridated at 0.7 to 1.2 mg/l – with a *Recommended Control Range* allowing 1.7 mg/l. Worse, school water systems could be fluoridated at levels up to 4.5 times higher than communities![23b]

In patients with fluorosis, the elastic properties of the ascending aorta are impaired.[24] Arterial stiffness precedes and contributes to the development of hypertension.[25] Significant increases in arterial stiffness were measured in women with preeclampsia compared with those with gestational hypertension.[25b] (See also page 77: Vascular Aging and Arterial Stiffness.)

In 2018, it was shown that arterial stiffness is inversely correlated with the diversity and abundance of microorganisms in the gut microbiome of women.[26] (See Chapter 3.)

Fluoride and Calcification in Arteries and the Pineal Gland
An increased prevalence of carotid artery atherosclerosis in adults is associated with increased levels of fluoride in drinking water.[27] In coronary arteries, fluoride uptake is considerably higher in patients with cardiovascular events. PET/CT scans show a significant correlation between fluoride uptake and calcification in most of arterial walls.[28] (Preeclampsia is a marker for women who will experience premature cardiovascular and cerebrovascular diseases.[29])

Fluoride and calcium concentrations are also positively related in the brain's pineal gland. The NRC said, "Fluoride is likely to cause decreased melatonin production and to have other effects on normal pineal function, which in turn could contribute to a variety of effects in humans."[30] (See Appendix B.)

Fluoride, Oxidative Stress, and Placental Melatonin
Oxidative stress is a recognized mode of fluoride toxicity that has been observed in several types of cells and also in different organ systems in animals and in people.[31]

Increasing oxidative stress in children with fluorosis is associated with increasing fluoride concentration in their drinking water.[32] Preeclamptic placentas exhibit a greater extent of both ER stress and oxidative stress.[33]

Melatonin is essential for proper trophoblastic function and development and has been shown to ameliorate oxidative damage to the placenta and to the fetus.[34,35] Furthermore, melatonin upregulates the antioxidant defense system impaired by fluoride-induced oxidative stress.[36]

In preeclampsia, maternal blood levels of melatonin are decreased. Lanoix et al. (2012) have shown that the human placenta produces melatonin and expresses its receptors. The researchers found that expression of melatonin receptors is significantly reduced in preeclamptic placentas.[37]

Melatonin has been described as a *suicidal* antioxidant. Once oxidized, it cannot be reduced to its former state.[38] By reacting with fluoride, the melatonin available to the placenta is reduced.

Acetaminophen and Fluoride – Synergistic Damage
Acetaminophen, the medication most commonly used by pregnant women for fevers and pain, is associated with an increased risk of preeclampsia when taken during the third trimester.[39]

Even at low doses, acetaminophen can cause oxidative stress,[40] but co-exposure with fluoride has a synergistic toxic effect. Together, acetaminophen and fluoride (in sub-toxic doses) enhance oxidative stress and kidney damage in rats, as compared to rats treated only with fluoride or with acetaminophen. Acetaminophen also significantly decreases urinary fluoride excretion, which is how the body rids itself of previously absorbed fluoride.[41]

Note: rodents more efficiently clear fluoride from their bodies. It takes over 10 times the amount of fluoride to cause fluorosis in a mouse than it does in a human, therefore rodent studies involving higher doses of fluoride are relevant to humans.[15]

Angiogenic Factors and Fluoride
During mid-gestation, the maternal uterine spiral arteries must be transformed into low-resistance, high-capacitance blood vessels that can provide increasing amounts of oxygen and nutrients to the growing fetus. Poor spiral artery remodeling due to an abnormal balance of proangiogenic and antiangiogenic factors causes the hypertension seen in preeclampsia.

The fetus secretes adrenomedullin, a proangiogenic vasodilator, into the placenta. In normal human pregnancies, adrenomedullin is elevated approximately 5-fold in the maternal plasma, but often blunted in pregnancies complicated by preeclampsia.[42] Sodium fluoride has been shown to completely block the effect of adrenomedullin in pregnant rats.[43]

Soluble endoglin (sEng) is an antiangiogenic protein whose levels are elevated in women with preeclampsia. Studies have identified sEng levels 4-fold higher in women with severe preeclampsia than in normal pregnancies.[44] In amniotic fluid, sEng concentrations were shown to be three times higher in preeclamptic, compared with uncomplicated pregnancies (1.9 vs 0.6 ng/ml).[45] When amniotic tissue cultures were treated with sodium fluoride, Tskitishvili et al. (2010) found significantly higher expression levels of sEng – at any dose and time tested.[46] sEng is a marker of endothelial dysfunction, a central mechanism in preeclampsia and diseases of aging. (Page 76.)

Fetal fluoride levels depend on maternal fluoride exposure. Cord blood fluoride concentrations doubled, when mothers consumed 1.5 mg of fluoride daily during their third trimester.[46b] When pregnant women consume 1.25 mg of fluoride per day, the fluoride concentration in their amniotic fluid is significantly higher than in women who consume 0.25–1.0 mg fluoride.[47] (Discussed on page 50: Fluoridated Amniotic Fluid)

Fluoride levels in amniotic fluid – which are considerably higher at term than earlier in the third trimester[48] – are positively correlated in a dose-response relationship with fluoride content and pathology of fetal bones, with significantly greater fluoride levels in fetuses born to mothers who have dental fluorosis.[49]

Inflammation: Periodontitis, Preeclampsia, and Dental Fluorosis
Maternal periodontal disease with systemic inflammation as measured by hs-CRP (high-sensitivity C-reactive protein) is increased in preeclampsia and represents a marker of its severity.[50,51]

Women with a history of periodontal treatment are more likely to develop severe preeclampsia than women without a prior history of treatment.[52] Periodontal treatment exposes women to extremely high concentrations of topical fluoride (22,600 ppm), some of which is absorbed into the bloodstream and placenta.

Plasma levels of hs-CRP are significantly higher among patients with fluorosis compared to controls.[53] A clinical study found a strong association of occurrence of periodontal disease in people who had dental fluorosis. As the severity of fluorosis increased, periodontitis increased from 8.5% to 35.8%. Also, periodontitis was significantly more common in females.[54] Many studies and published documents have shown that increased fluoride exposure is directly linked to increased periodontal disease.[55]

Elevated liver enzymes, an inflammatory factor in preeclampsia, is significantly higher in early-onset preeclampsia.[56] In children, elevated liver enzymes have been correlated with the levels of fluoride in their drinking water (in a dose-response manner) and with the degree of fluorosis in their teeth.[57]

Preeclampsia Increases Risk of Autism and Preterm Birth
Preeclampsia increases the risk of having a child with autism spectrum disorder, and risk increases with greater preeclampsia severity. (See page 58.) Furthermore, autism spectrum disorder is related to ER stress.[58]

Preeclamptic women with periodontal disease are at greater risk for preterm delivery.[59] Preeclampsia is the underlying cause of about 25% of all medically indicated preterm deliveries. As discussed in Chapter 1, prenatal fluoride is a risk factor for preterm birth.

Fluoridated Water, Dental Fluorosis, and Preeclampsia
A case-control study found a significant association between fluoride levels in drinking water, dental fluorosis in mothers, and low birthweight of newborns. Preeclampsia was significantly associated with low birthweight (23.1% in cases vs. 11.6% in controls).[60]

Systemic exposure to fluoride through drinking water is associated with an increased risk of dental and bone fluorosis in a dose-response manner, without a detectable threshold.[61] British researchers estimate the prevalence of dental fluorosis of all levels of severity to be 15% in nonfluoridated areas and 48% in fluoridated areas.[62]

In the US from 1987 to 2004, the prevalence of moderate and severe dental fluorosis nearly tripled from 1.3% to 3.6%.[63] There was also a 13.7% increase in the percentage of Americans receiving public water that was fluoridated (from 60.5% to 68.8%).[64]

During the same 18 years, the incidence rate of preeclampsia rose by 25%: from 23.6 to 29.4 cases per 1,000 deliveries.[65] Rates of severe pre-eclampsia are steadily increasing. In the largest US cohort study (120 million births), the prevalence rate for severe preeclampsia increased 5 times: from 0.3% in 1980 to 1.4% in 2010.[29]

The available population data reveal that in the two most fluoridated US regions (South and Northeast) from 1996–2004, the preeclampsia rate averaged 19% higher than in the two least fluoridated regions (Midwest and West): 31.7 vs. 26.6 cases per 1,000 deliveries.

The preeclampsia rate averaged 40% higher in the South than in the West: 34.1 vs. 24.3 cases per 1,000 deliveries.[65] In 2004, the average fluoridation rate in the South's 16 states was 81%, compared to 46% in the West's 13 states.

Note: In the 22 states that were fluoridated at 80% or more (average 92%), the age-adjusted death rate (2010) for essential hypertension and hypertensive renal disease was 9% higher than in the 27 states fluoridated at less than 80% (average 56%).[66]

Fluoridated Water, Hypothyroidism, and Preeclampsia
In 2015, a major population-level study analyzed data from 99% of England's 8,020 general medical practices. It found a positive association between fluoride levels in water and patients diagnosed with hypothyroidism. High hypothyroidism prevalence was 30% more likely in practices located in areas with fluoride levels in excess of 0.3 mg/l. Those located in the West Midlands (a wholly fluoridated area) were nearly twice as likely to report high hypothyroidism prevalence in comparison with Greater Manchester (nonfluoridated area).[67] The study did not include undiagnosed subclinical hypothyroidism.

Preeclampsia is often complicated by subclinical hypothyroidism. Many studies have shown a relation between the level of thyroid hormones and development and severity of preeclampsia.[68] In an analysis of pregnancy outcomes in 24,883 women, there was a significant association between subclinical hypothyroidism and severe preeclampsia.[69] A 2013 retrospective cohort study of 223,512 pregnancies found that primary hypothyroidism was associated with increased odds of preeclampsia.[70]

Singh et al. (2014) tested drinking water and body fluids for fluoride content plus thyroid hormone levels in children with dental fluorosis. "Different degrees of dental fluorosis could be observed, with significant deviation in the serum thyroid hormone levels."[71] Note: ER stress has been detected in the thyroid glands of fetuses whose mothers had dental fluorosis.[17]

Hypothyroidism is associated with ADHD and is considered a potential cause of the disorder. Also published in 2015 was the first population-based study to examine the relationship between exposure to fluoridated water and ADHD prevalence. A multivariate regression analysis showed that artificial water fluoridation prevalence was significantly positively associated with ADHD prevalence. After socioeconomic status was controlled, each 1% increase in artificial fluoridation prevalence in 1992 was associated with about 67,000 to 131,000 additional ADHD diagnoses from 2003 to 2011 in the US.[72] (See p. 59: Fluoridated Water: Hypothyroidism, Autism and ADHD)

FDA: Fluoride and Pregnancy
The FDA classified fluoride as an unapproved drug in Pregnancy Category C: "Animal reproduction studies have shown an adverse effect on the fetus, and there are no adequate and well-controlled studies in humans." The FDA warns that a drug in category C "may pose risks similar to a drug in Category X,"[73] which carries the warning: "The risks involved in use of the drug in pregnant women clearly outweigh potential benefits."

As for any potential benefits of swallowing fluoride, after reviewing the best available evidence for the effectiveness of water fluoridation, the FDA would only allow a very weak claim: "Drinking fluoridated water may reduce the risk of tooth decay."[74] *May reduce risk* is a far cry from reduces tooth decay 40 to 65% – the longtime sales pitch of fluoridation promoters.[75] Drinking pure water also may reduce the risk of tooth decay. (See Appendix D.)

Since 1966, the FDA has prohibited claims that prenatal fluoride supplements benefit the teeth of children.[76] The US Centers for Disease Control and Prevention has "good evidence to reject the use" of fluoride supplements for pregnant women. Furthermore, "No published studies confirm the effectiveness of fluoride supplements in controlling dental caries among persons ages >16 years."[77]

Fluoridation chemicals (increasingly from China) are intentionally added to about 75% of US tap water. An EPA-regulated "water contaminant," fluoride now pervades the nation's processed food and beverage chain, essentially making the US *artificially fluoride endemic*. The amount of fluoride people consume is unknown, because fluoride content is not stated on labels, even though the National Research Council said they should be. (See Appendix B.)

Research Needed
For women who previously experienced preeclampsia, determine if their drinking water was fluoridated. Did they regularly drink tea or beverages manufactured with fluoridated water? How severe was their preeclampsia? Do they have dental fluorosis, a biomarker of their genetic susceptibility to fluoride?

A next step: Compare the concentration of fluoride in preeclamptic placentas with the severity of preeclampsia, as well as with placentas from normal pregnancies. It should be standard procedure to measure fluoride levels in blood and urine prior to and during pregnancy. Measuring arterial stiffness would also be useful in predicting preeclampsia.[25b]

> "Fluoride has no known essential function in human growth and development and no signs of fluoride deficiency have been identified." – European Food Safety Authority.[7]

Preventing Preeclampsia
Preeclampsia used to be called "toxemia," until 20th-century science failed to identify the causative toxin. The current name *preeclampsia* (pre-convulsions) continues to reflect the failure to determine the etiology of this life-threatening disease of the placenta.

This century's science reveals that a far more
accurate term for preeclampsia is *placental fluorosis*.

Bottom line: Not ingesting fluoride poses absolutely no risk (or lack of benefit) to the placenta or fetus; however, consumption of fluoride may very well increase the risk of preeclampsia and its dangerous short-term and lifelong consequences for mother and child.

Mothers-to-be should not swallow fluoride in supplements, in dental products, or during dental procedures. They should not consume fluoridated water or beverages manufactured with it.

References – Placental Fluorosis: Fluoride and Preeclampsia

1. Jido TA, Yakasai IA. Preeclampsia: a review of the evidence. *Ann Afr Med.* 2013 Apr-Jun;12(2):75–85.

2. Preeclampsia Foundation. FAQs and Preeclampsia Fact Sheet. Accessed June 26, 2018.

3. Gardner DE, Smith FA, Hodge HC, Overton DE, Feltman R. The fluoride concentration of placental tissue as related to fluoride content in drinking water. *Science.* 1952;115(2982):208–209.

4. Chlubek D, Poreba R, Machalinski B. Fluoride and calcium distribution in human placenta. *Fluoride.* 1998 31(3):131–136.

   Gurumurthy SM, Mohanty S, Rao P. Role of placenta to combat fluorosis (in fetus) in endemic fluorosis area. *Natl J Integr Res Med.* 2010 Oct–Dec;1(4):16–19.

5. Williams PJ, Pipkin FB. The genetics of pre-eclampsia and other hypertensive disorders of pregnancy. *Best Pract Res Clin Obstet Gynaecol.* 2011 Aug;25(4-4):405–417.

6. Everett ET. Fluoride's effects on the formation of teeth and bones, and the influence of genetics. *J Dent Res.* 2011 May;90(5):552–560.

7. European Food Safety Authority. Scientific Opinion on Dietary Reference Values for Fluoride. *EFSA J.* 2013;11(8):3332.

8. Connett M. Racial disparities in dental fluorosis. Fluoride Action Network. June 2012.

9. Preeclampsia strikes African Americans women hard. Preeclampsia Foundation. January 31, 2013.

10. Breathett K, Muhlestein D, Foraker R, Gulati M. Differences in preeclampsia rates between African American and Caucasian women: trends from the National Hospital Discharge Survey. *J Womens Health (Larchmt).* 2014 Nov;23(11):886–893.

11. Agalakova NI, Gusev GP. Molecular mechanisms of cytotoxicity and apoptosis induced by inorganic fluoride. *ISRN Cell Biol.* 2012:403835.

12. Pincus D, Aranda-Díaz A, Zuleta IA, Walter P, El-Samad H. Delayed Ras/PKA signaling augments the unfolded protein response. *Proc Natl Acad Sci USA.* 2014 Oct14;111(41):14800–14805.

13. Yoshida H. ER stress and diseases. *FEBS J.* 2007 Feb;274(3):630–658.

14. Buhimschi IA, Nayeri UA, Zhao G, et al. Protein misfolding, congophilia, oligomerization, and defective amyloid processing in preeclampsia. *Sci Transl Med*. 2014 Jul;16(245):245ra92.

15. Sharma R, Tsuchiya M, Bartlett JD. Fluoride induces endoplasmic reticulum stress and inhibits protein synthesis and secretion. *Environ Health Perspect*. 2008 Sep;116(9):1142–1146.

16. National Research Council. *Fluoride in drinking water: A scientific review of EPA's standards*. National Academies Press; 2006:178.

17. Zhou YL, Shi HY, Li XN, et al. Role of endoplasmic reticulum stress in aberrant activation of fluoride-treated osteoblasts. *Biol Trace Elem Res*. 2013 Sep;154(3):448–456.

18. Saad El-Dien HM, El Gamal DA, Mubarak HA, Saleh SM. Effect of fluoride on rat cerebellar cortex: light and electron microscopic studies. *Egypt J Histol*. 2010 June;33(2):245–256.

19. He H, Cheng Z, Liu W. The effects of fluorine on the human fetus. *Fluoride*. 2008 Oct–Dec;41(4):321–326.

20. Yanni YU. Effects of fluoride on the ultrastructure of glandular epithelial cells of human fetuses. *Chin J Epidemiology*. 2000 Mar;19(2):81–83.

20b. Kliman HJ. 2006. From trophoblast to human placenta (from The Encyclopedia of Reproduction). Yale University School of Medicine.

21. Burton GJ, Yung HW. Endoplasmic reticulum stress in the pathogenesis of early-onset preeclampsia. *Pregnancy Hypertens*. 2011 Jan;1(1-2):72–78.

22. Varol E, Varol S. Water-borne fluoride and primary hypertension. *Fluoride*. 2013 Jan–Mar; 46(1)3–6.

23. Sun L, Gao Y, Liu H, et al. An assessment of the relationship between excess fluoride intake from drinking water and essential hypertension in adults residing in fluoride endemic areas. *Total Environ*. 2013 Jan 15;443:864–869.

23b. Centers for Disease Control and Prevention. *Fluoridation Census 1989*. July 1991. Table A: School Systems. Page iii.

24. Varol E, Akcay S, Ersoy IH, Ozaydin M, Koroglu BK, Varol S. Aortic elasticity is impaired in patients with endemic fluorosis. *Biol Trace Elem Res*. 2010 Feb;133(2):121–127.

25. Mitchell GF. Recent advances in hypertension: Arterial stiffness and hypertension. *Hypertension*. 2014 Jul;64(1):13–18.

25b. Hausvater A, Giannone T, Sandoval YH, et al. The association between preeclampsia and arterial stiffness. *J Hypertens*. 2012 Jan;30(1):17–33.

26. Menni C, Lin C, Cecelja M, et al. Gut microbial diversity is associated with lower arterial stiffness in women. *Eur Heart J*. 2018; 39:2390–7.

27. Liu H, Gao Y, Sun L, Li M, Li B, Sun D. Assessment of relationship on excess fluoride intake from drinking water and carotid atherosclerosis development in adults in fluoride endemic areas, China. *Int J Hyg Environ Health*. 2014 Mar;217(2–3):413–420.

28. Li Y, Berenji GR, Shaba WF, Tafti B, Yevdayev E, Dadparvar S. Association of vascular fluoride uptake with vascular calcification and coronary artery disease. *Nucl Med Commun*. 2012 Jan;33(1):14–20.

    Bank T. Fluoride & Arterial Calcification. Fluoride Action Network. July 2012.

29. Ananth CV, Keyes KM, Wapner RJ. Pre-eclampsia rates in the United States, 1980–2010: age-period-cohort analysis. *BMJ*. 2013;347:f6564.

30. National Research Council. Op cit., 253, 256.

31. Barbier O, Arreola-Mendoza L, Del Razo LM. Molecular mechanisms of fluoride toxicity. *Chem Biol Interact*. 2010 Nov 5;188(2):319–333.

32. Ailani V, Gupta RC, Gupta SK, Gupta K. Oxidative stress in cases of chronic fluoride intoxication. *Indian J Clin Biochem*. 2009 Oct;24(4): 426-29.

33. Burton GJ, Yung HW, Cindrova-Davies T, Charnock-Jones DS. Placental endoplasmic reticulum stress and oxidative stress in the pathophysiology of unexplained intrauterine growth restriction and early onset preeclampsia. *Placenta*. 2009 Mar;30 Suppl A:S43–48.

34. Sagrillo-Fagundes L, Soliman A, Vaillancourt C. Maternal and placental melatonin: actions and implication for successful pregnancies. *Minerva Ginecol*. 2014 Jun;66(3):251–266.

35. Reiter RJ, Tan DX, Korkmaz A, Rosales-Corral SA. Melatonin and stable circadian rhythms optimize maternal, placental and fetal physiology. *Hum Reprod Update*. 2014 Mar–Apr;20(2):293–307.

36. Bharti VK, Srivastava RS, Kumar H, et al. Effects of melatonin and epiphyseal proteins on fluoride-induced adverse changes in antioxidant status of heart, liver, and kidney of rats. *Adv Pharmacol Sci*. Volume 2014 (2014), Article ID 532969.

37. Lanoix D, Guérin P, Vaillancourt C. Placental melatonin production and melatonin receptor expression are altered in preeclampsia: new insights into the role of this hormone in pregnancy. *J Pineal Res.* 2012 Nov;53(4):417-25.

38. Lobo V, Patil A, Phatak A, Chandra N. Free radicals, antioxidants and functional foods: impact on human health. *Pharmacogn Rev.* 2010 Jul–Dec; 4(8):118–126.

39. Rebordosa C, Zelop CM, Kogevinas M, Sørensen HT, Olsen J. Use of acetaminophen during pregnancy and risk of preeclampsia, hypertensive and vascular disorders: a birth cohort study. *J Matern Fetal Neonatal Med.* 2010 May;23(5):371–378.

40. Bauer AZ, Kriebel D. Prenatal and perinatal analgesic exposure and autism: an ecological link. *Environ Health.* 2013;12:41.

41. Inkielewicz-Stępniak I, Knap N. Effect of exposure to fluoride and acetaminophen on oxidative/nitrosative status of liver and kidney in male and female rats. *Pharmacol Rep.* 2012;64(4):902–911.

42. Li M, Schwerbrock NM, Lenhart PM, et al. Fetal-derived adrenomedullin mediates the innate immune milieu of the placenta. *J Clin Invest.* 2013 Jun;123(6):2408–2420.

   Hughes T. Baby knows best: fetuses emit hormone crucial to preventing preeclampsia. University of North Carolina Health Care. May 1, 2013.

43. Ross GR, Yallampalli U, Yallampalli C. Cyclic AMP-independent CGRP8-37-sensitive receptors mediate adrenomedullin-induced decrease of CaCl2-contraction in pregnant rat mesenteric artery. *J Vasc Res.* 2008; 45(1):33–44.

44. Al-Jameil N. A brief overview of preeclampsia. *J Clin Med Res.* 2014 February; 6(1): 1–7.

45. Staff AC, Braekke K, Johnsen GM, Karumanchi SA, Harsem NK. Circulating concentrations of soluble endoglin (CD105) in fetal and maternal serum and in amniotic fluid in preeclampsia. *Am J Obstet Gynecol.* 2007 Aug;197(2):176.e1–6.

46. Tskitishvili E, Sharentuya N, Temma-Asano K, et al. Oxidative stress-induced S100B protein from placenta and amnion affects soluble endoglin release from endothelial cells. *Mol Hum Reprod.* 2010;16(3):188–199. Figures 5C, 5D.

46b. Caldera R, Chavinie J, Fermanian J, et al. Maternal-fetal transfer of fluoride in pregnant women. *Biol Neonate.* 1988;54(5):263–269.

47. Brambilla E, Belluomo G, Malerba A, Buscaglia M, Strohmenger L. Oral administration of fluoride in pregnant women, and the relation between concentration in maternal plasma and in amniotic fluid. *Arch Oral Biol.* 1994 Nov;39(11):991–994.

48. Chlubek D, Mokrzyński S, Machoy Z, Olszewska M. Fluorides in the body of the mother and in the fetus. III. Fluorides in amniotic fluid. *Ginekol Pol.* 1995 Nov;66(11):614–617.

49. Shi J, Dai G, Zhang Z. Relationship between bone fluoride content, pathological change in bone of aborted fetuses and maternal fluoride level. *Zhonghua Yu Fang Yi Xue Za Zhi.* 1995 Mar;29(2):103–105.

50. Mihu D, Costin N, Mihu CM, Blaga LD, Pop RB. C-reactive protein, marker for evaluation of systemic inflammatory response in preeclampsia. *Rev Med Chir Soc Med Nat Iasi.* 2008 Oct–Dec;112(4):1019–1025.

51. Ruma M, Boggess K, Moss K, et al. Maternal periodontal disease, systemic inflammation, and risk for preeclampsia. *Am J Obstet Gynecol.* 2008 Apr;198(4):389.e1–5.

52. Boggess KA, Berggren EK, Koskenoja V, Urlaub D, Lorenz C. Severe preeclampsia and maternal self-report of oral health, hygiene, and dental care. *J Periodontol.* 2013 Feb;84(2):143–151.

53. Varol E, Aksoy F, Icli A, et al. Increased plasma neopterin and hs-CRP levels in patients with endemic fluorosis. *Bull Environ Contam Toxicol.* 2012 Nov;89(5):931–936.

54. Vandana KL, Reddy MS. Assessment of periodontal status in dental fluorosis subjects using community periodontal index of treatment needs. *Indian J Dent Res.* 2007 Apr–Jun;18(2):67–71.

55. Waugh D. Fluoride exposure and periodontal disease. Enviro Management Services. 2012.

56. Peraçoli JC, Bannwart-Castro CF, Romao M, et al. High levels of heat shock protein 70 are associated with pro-inflammatory cytokines and may differentiate early- from late-onset preeclampsia. *J Reprod Immunol.* 2013 Dec;100(2):129–134.

57. Xiong X, Liu J, He W, et al. Dose-effect relationship between drinking water fluoride levels and damage to liver and kidney functions in children. *Environ Res.* 2007 Jan;103(1):112–116.

58. Fujita E, Dai H, Tanabe Y, et al. Autism spectrum disorder is related to endoplasmic reticulum stress induced by mutations in the synaptic cell adhesion molecule, CADM1. *Cell Death Dis.* 2010 Jun;1(6):e47.

59. Pattanashetti JI, NagathanVM, Rao SM. Evaluation of periodontitis as a risk for preterm birth among preeclamptic and non-preeclamptic pregnant women – a case control study. *J Clin Diagn Res*. 2013 Aug;7(8):1776–1778.

60. Diouf M, Cisse D, Lo CM, Ly M, Faye D, Ndiaye O. Pregnant women living in areas of endemic fluorosis in Senegal and low birthweight newborns: case-control study. *Rev Epidemiol Sante Publique*. 2012 Apr; 60(2):103–108. Translation of full study.

61. Scientific Committee on Health and Environmental Risks (SCHER). Critical review of any new evidence on the hazard profile, health effects, and human exposure to fluoride and the fluoridating agents of drinking water. European Commission. May 16, 2011. Abstract.

62. British Fluoridation Society. Dental fluorosis. *One in a Million: the facts about water fluoridation*. 2012.

63. Beltrán-Aguilar ED, Barker L, Dye BA. Prevalence and severity of dental fluorosis in the United States, 1999–2004. *NCHS Data Brief*. 2010 Nov;(53):1–8.

64. Centers for Disease Control and Prevention (CDC). Fluoridation growth.

65. Wallis AB, Saftlas AF, Hsia J, Atrash HK. Secular trends in the rates of preeclampsia, eclampsia, and gestational hypertension, United States, 1987–2004. *Am J Hypertens*. 2008 May;21(5):521–526. Full study.

66. Murphy SL, Xu J, Kochanek KD. Deaths: Final data for 2010. *National Vital Statistics Reports*. 2013 May8;61(4):86.

67. Peckham S, Lowery D, Spencer S. Are fluoride levels in drinking water associated with hypothyroidism prevalence in England? A large observational study of GP practice data and fluoride levels in drinking water. *J Epidemiol Community Health*. 2015;0:1–6.

68. Raoofi Z, Jalilian A, Zanjani MS, Parvar SP, Parvar SP. Comparison of thyroid hormone levels between normal and preeclamptic pregnancies. *Med J Islam Repub Iran*. 2014;28:1.

69. Wilson KL, Casey BM, McIntire DD, Halvorson LM, Cunningham FG. Subclinical thyroid disease and the incidence of hypertension in pregnancy. *Obstet Gynecol*. 2012 Feb;119(2 Pt 1):315–320.

70. Männistö T, Mendola P, Grewal J, Xie Y, Chen Z, Laughon SK. Thyroid diseases and adverse pregnancy outcomes in a contemporary US cohort. *J Clin Endocrinol Metab*. 2013 Jul;98(7):2725–2733.

71. Singh N, Verma KG, Verma P, Sidhu GK, Sachdeva S. A comparative study of fluoride ingestion levels, serum thyroid hormone & TSH level derangements, dental fluorosis status among school children from endemic and non-endemic fluorosis areas. *Springerplus*. 2014;3:7.

72. Malin AJ, Till C. Exposure to fluoridated water and attention deficit hyperactivity disorder prevalence among children and adolescents in the United States: an ecological association. *Environ Health*. 2015;14:17.

73. US Food and Drug Administration. Summary of proposed rule on pregnancy and lactation labeling. *Federal Register*. 2008 May29;73(104): 30833-34.

74. Food and Drug Administration. Health claim notification for fluoridated water and reduced risk of dental caries. 2006.

75. Hileman B. Fluoridation of water: Questions about health risks and benefits remain after more than 40 years. *Chem Eng News*. August 1, 1988. Page 27.

76. Institute of Medicine. *Dietary reference intakes for calcium, phosphorus, magnesium, vitamin D, and fluoride*. Washington, DC: National Academies Press; 1997:304.

77. US Centers for Disease Control and Prevention. Recommendations for using fluoride to prevent and control dental caries in the United States. *Morb Mortal Rep*. August 17, 2001;50(14);3. Table 4 (footnote).

Chapter 3

Fluoride swallowed in amniotic fluid may disrupt
colonization and composition of bacteria in the fetal GI tract –
adversely affecting immunological and neurological development.

An earlier version of this report was
published in the April 2016 *Townsend Letter:
The Examiner of Alternative Medicine*

Prenatal Fluoride and Autism

Increasing evidence reveals that prenatal exposures to some widely used chemicals are implicated in the growing pandemic of developmental neurotoxicity.[1,2] Fluoride is the most controversial of these chemicals, because it is the only one intentionally added to the water consumed by more than 200 million Americans, including pregnant women and their unborn children.

Topical fluoride in toothpaste has been used since the 1950s to reduce tooth decay. A primary mechanism of fluoride's ability to prevent dental caries is its strong antimicrobial effects. It is well established that fluoride can inhibit the growth of bacteria, says Robert Breaker, PhD, a National Academy of Sciences award-winning molecular biologist. He admits, however, "There has been little understanding of its precise effects on cells."[3] (See pages 7-8.)

Fluoride Weakens Bacterial Adhesion Forces

In 2013, a key antimicrobial mechanism of fluoride was identified by researchers in experimental physics at Saarland University in Germany. Using artificial tooth surfaces (hydroxyapatite pellets), they tested fluoride's effect on the adhesion forces of cariogenic bacteria (*Streptococcus mutans* and *Streptococcus oralis*), including a non-pathogenic bacterium (*Staphylococcus carnosus*).

After they were exposed to fluoride, atomic force microscopy revealed that all three bacteria species exhibited lower adhesion forces. Because fluoride makes bacteria less able to stick to teeth, decay-causing microorganisms are more easily washed away by saliva or brushing. The researchers said, "Fluoride appears to weaken bacterial adhesion forces in general."[4,5]

This raises the question: How do weakened bacterial adhesion forces affect the developing gastrointestinal tract, whose vast and complex ecosystem – collectively called the gut microbiota or microbiome – plays an essential role in neurological and immunological development and health?

Adhesion Forces and Bacterial Colonization of the GI Tract

The process of surface adhesion is a survival strategy employed by virtually all bacteria and refined over millions of years.[6] Adhesion of bacteria to intestinal mucosa is often recognized as a prerequisite for microbial colonization of the human gastrointestinal (GI) tract.[7] Emerging research shows this process begins in the womb.[8-11]

Distinct microbial populations have recently been discovered at maternal sites that were previously thought to be sterile, including the amniotic cavity and meconium (first feces of a newborn infant). Our understanding of the impact of fetal microbial contact on health outcomes is still rudimentary.[12]

Of the many potential sources for a prenatal microbiome, amniotic fluid flora accounted for the greater relative abundance of bacteria found in meconium than either the oral or vaginal cavities of pregnant women.[13,14] When pregnant women consumed specific probiotics, microbial DNA in their amniotic fluid was associated with changes in gene expression in the fetal intestine.[15]

Fluoridated Amniotic Fluid
Amniotic fluid is arguably our most precious bodily fluid. Early in the second trimester, a fetus begins swallowing amniotic fluid, which passes through its digestive system and kidneys, is excreted as urine, then swallowed again – recycling the full volume of amniotic fluid every few hours. By the time the child is born, up to 15 ounces of amniotic fluid are consumed per day.

Fetal swallowing contributes importantly to gastrointestinal development as a result of the large volume of ingested fluid. Nutrients, hormones, and growth factors in amniotic fluid bathing the fetal intestine during the third trimester are needed to produce a profound maturational effect on the intestine's ability to appropriately respond to colonizing bacteria.[16]

Fluoride concentrations in human amniotic fluid are about 50% of maternal serum levels and are considerably higher at term than earlier in pregnancy.[17,18] Women who consumed 1.25 mg of fluoride per day had a significantly higher fluoride concentration in their amniotic fluid than women who consumed 0.25 to 1.0 mg per day.[19] Note: the US Institute of Medicine says the recommended Adequate Intake (AI) of fluoride for pregnant women is 3 mg per day.[20]

The fluoride concentration in women's amniotic fluid was 0.017 mg/l, when their drinking water contained <0.5 mg/l of fluoride.[18] A similar fluoride concentration is secreted by salivary glands into the ductal saliva of children who drink fluoridated water.[21] This very low level of fluoride provides the "systemic" benefit, the primary rationale for swallowing fluoride in water.

A low concentration of fluoride that is continually swallowed and recycled in amniotic fluid must also be bioactive in the fetal GI tract.

In fact, a primary reason why pregnant women are told to consume fluoridated water is to delay bacterial colonization in their baby.[22]

> The American Academy of Pediatric Dentistry encourages perinatal fluoride exposure to help "delay colonisation of the infant oral cavity by cariogenic bacteria." [22]
> – *Health Effects of Water Fluoridation*
> *a Review of the Scientific Evidence* (New Zealand)

Altered Microbiome in Autism Spectrum Disorder
Antimicrobials, including low-dose antimicrobials in food and water supplies, indiscriminately affect all members of the gut microbial ecosystem, especially decreasing the levels of beneficial bifidobacteria and increasing the levels of potentially harmful clostridia, as seen in the microbiota of autistic children.[23,24]

Autism is closely associated with a distinct gut microflora that can be characterized by reduced richness and diversity as well as by altered composition and structure of the microbial community; specifically, lower levels of important groups of carbohydrate-degrading or fermenting microbes.[24-28]

In a rodent model for autism spectrum disorder (ASD), autism-like behavior is associated with altered microbial colonization and activity.[29] These mice have abnormally low levels of *Bacteroides fragilis*, a bacterium that modulates levels of several metabolites and is one of the earliest-colonizing and most abundant microbes in a healthy human intestinal tract.[30] Feeding *B. fragilis* to these mice ameliorates defects in communicative, repetitive, and anxiety-like behaviors.[31]

Gut Bacteria, Immune System, Autism, and Fluoride
Increasing evidence indicates that the gut microbiota influences the immune and nervous systems and vice versa.[32] Microbial contact *in utero* is associated with changes in fetal intestinal innate immune gene expression profile.[15] (See page 62 for a 2018 research update.)

The GI tract has 70 to 80% of the body's immune cells and is the primary site of interaction between the immune system and microorganisms, both symbiotic and pathogenic.[33] Proper microbial colonization and composition of the GI tract are essential for the maturation of the immune system.[8,23,34,35] Different bacteria have clearly defined adherence sites and immunological effects.[36] Immune system dysregulation in autism has been reported in several studies.[37]

During colonization of the gut with *B. fragilis*, the cellular and physical maturation of the developing immune system is directed by a bacterial polysaccharide.[30] Ochoa-Repáraz et al. (2010) found that a polysaccharide of *B. fragilis* can protect against central nervous system demyelinating disease.[38] Human and animal studies implicate impairments of myelination in autism.[39,40]

Sodium fluoride has been shown to reduce bacterial polysaccharide production by inhibiting bacterial attachment.[41] A mechanism of action for fluoride's ability to reduce bacterial adhesion forces is its inhibitory effect on the activity of glucan-binding proteins.[42] In the GI tract, glucans represent a significant potential in the suppression or treatment of several gastrointestinal problems.[43]

Adhesion Molecules, Autism, and Fluoride
In its very comprehensive 2006 report, *Fluoride in Drinking Water: A Scientific Review of EPA's Standards*, the US National Research Council concluded, "It is apparent that fluorides have the ability to interfere with the functions of the brain and the body by direct and indirect means."[44] (See Appendix B.)

Fluoride's indirect effects on neurodevelopment via the fetal microbiome have yet to be researched, however, evidence is growing for fluoride's direct effects on the fetal brain. Fluoride concentrations in brain tissue are about "20% of plasma" and possibly "higher for exposure before development of the blood-brain barrier."[45]

Autism involves early brain overgrowth and dysfunction, an excess of neurons in the prefrontal cortex caused by a prenatal disruption of developing brain architecture as early as the second trimester.[46] Research by Lahiri et al. (2013) suggests that brain enlargement in autism is likely due to cell adhesion dysfunction.[47]

Neural cell adhesion molecules (NCAM) are widely expressed in the nervous system, where they are involved in axon growth and guidance – fundamental processes that underlie formation of the synaptic connections and myelinated nerve structure crucial to brain development.

Significantly lower serum levels of several types of adhesion molecules, including NCAM, have been found in ASD.[48,49] Neural pathways involving synaptic cell adhesion are disrupted in some people with autism, including alterations in the structure and expression of NCAM.[50,51]

Fluoride exposure has been shown to cause a dose-dependent decrease in NCAM expression levels in rat hippocampal neurons. In particular, the NCAM-140 protein expression level was significantly lower in response to the lowest dose of fluoride used.[52,53] NCAM-140 is found in migrating growth cones that are crucial to the formation of synaptic connections.[54]

Fluoride Adversely Affects Synaptic Development
ASD and Alzheimer's are increasingly being linked to defects in the organization and number of synapses, the tens of trillions of tiny yet complex structures that link neurons so they can communicate with each other. A molecule that helps create and maintain the scaffolding around which a synapse is built is postsynaptic density protein-95 (PSD-95). Neuronal synapses with less PSD-95 are likely to be weakened or lost.[55]

PSD-95 is concentrated at synapses where it regulates adhesion and enhances maturation of the presynaptic terminal. Research demonstrates that PSD-95 orchestrates synaptic development and plays an important role in synapse stabilization and plasticity.[56]

In rats that drank water with added fluoride for several months, the fluidity of brain synaptic membranes and the expression level of PSD-95 decreased in a dose-dependent manner.[57,58]

Rats anesthetized for 4 hours with 2.5% sevoflurane, a fluoride-based anesthetic, showed long-term deficits in hippocampal function and decreased hippocampal PSD-95 expression. "These data suggest that sevoflurane causes neurotoxicity in the developing brain."[56] In humans, exposure to 2.4% sevoflurane significantly increases serum fluoride levels.[59] (Sevoflurane is the most prevalent volatile anesthetic in pediatric anesthesia.)

Fluoride is a "Developmental Neurotoxicant"
In 2009, a team of researchers at the EPA's Neurotoxicology Division found *substantial evidence* that fluoride is one of 107 chemicals shown to be "toxic to the developing mammalian nervous system." Other *developmental neurotoxicants* on the list with fluoride are substances pregnant women already should avoid: Amphetamine, Arsenic, Bisphenol A, Chlorpyrifos, Cocaine, Ethanol (Alcohol), Lead, Mercury, Nicotine, Thalidomide, Valproate. (List is on page 2.)

In 2015, those researchers said fluoride is one of 22 *gold standard* substances "well documented to alter human neurodevelopment."[61] (Some of them, including fluoride, are also suspected in autism.[61b])

Fluoridation promoters say not to worry because "dose makes the poison," and the recommended level of fluoride in US drinking water is merely 0.7 mg/l (a concentration, not a dose). When it comes to neurodevelopment, however, a toxic substance's capacity to disrupt the developing brain is not simply dose dependent. It also depends on the "duration of exposure, and most important, on the timing during the developmental process," says the National Scientific Council on the Developing Child.[62]

> *A toxic substance's capacity to disrupt the developing brain depends, **most important, on the timing** during the developmental process.*[62]

When a Pregnant Woman Consumes Fluoride, So Does Her Baby
For ethical reasons, it is not feasible to measure fluoride levels in the bodies or brains of babies *in utero*. Instead, umbilical cord blood is readily obtained. Research shows that "fluoride levels in cord blood reach, on average, 87% (~60-90%) of those in maternal blood."[22]

Fetal blood fluoride levels, however, have been found to be twice as high as cord blood – and 25% higher than maternal concentrations.[63] As discussed above, this happens because babies in the womb swallow amniotic fluid which contains fluoride that is absorbed into fetal circulation[64] (as alcohol is[65]).

> Women have "significantly higher" fluoride levels in their amniotic fluid, when they consume 1.25 mg/day of fluoride[19] – the dose in about 8 cups of fluoridated US tap water.

Health authorities ignore fetal fluoride exposure, so safety thresholds are unknown. But the ones for children show that fetuses are exposed to unsafe levels of fluoride because of fluoridated water.

Tolerable Upper Intake Level of Fluoride
Safety thresholds are based on daily "Intake Levels" measured in milligrams per kilogram of body weight. In 1997, the US Institute of Medicine (IOM) established 0.10 mg/kg/day as the *Tolerable Upper Intake Level* (UL) of fluoride for children under 9 years old.[66]

A fetal UL was not determined, but it would be "significantly lower," said the IOM, because in the fetus, "sensitivity increases due to active placental transfer, accumulation of certain nutrients in the amniotic fluid, and rapid development of the brain."[67]

54

Fetuses are significantly more vulnerable to neurotoxins, so a fetal UL that is significantly lower than 0.10 mg/kg/day would reasonably be at a fifth of that: 0.02 mg/kg/day. This is comparable to the fluoride intake that 3rd-trimester babies receive daily when their mothers drink 8 cups of optimally fluoridated US tap water, as health authorities recommend. (See Appendix A.)

This suggests that in communities where tap water is fluoridated, babies in the womb are being exposed to fluoride at their Tolerable Upper Intake Level. According to the Institute of Medicine (2000):

> "A population mean intake at the UL suggests that as much as half of the population is consuming levels above the UL. **This would represent a very serious population risk of adverse effects.**"[68]

Poison Warning on Fluoride Toothpaste

Since 1997, the FDA has warned parents to: "Get medical help or contact a Poison Control Center right away" if a young child swallows more than a pea-sized dab of toothpaste that contains 0.25 mg of fluoride.

If a 5-year old swallows that much toothpaste, his *one-time* intake level of fluoride is about 0.01 mg/kg. A 3rd-trimester baby's *daily* fluoride intake level is comparable to that 5-year old's, when a pregnant woman drinks 4 cups of optimally fluoridated tap water. (See Appendix A.)

> With every 4 cups of fluoridated water a pregnant woman drinks, her baby's fluoride *intake level* is comparable to a child's who swallows too much fluoride in toothpaste.
>
> But instead of an FDA poison warning like fluoride toothpaste has, mothers-to-be are advised to drink 8 cups of fluoridated water every day!

The IOM said, "As intake increases above the UL, the risk of adverse effects increases,"[69] An *adverse effect* includes "any impairment of a physiologically important function."[70] Fluoridation promoters say not to worry because the IOM's *critical* adverse effect for children is moderate enamel fluorosis, "a cosmetic effect rather than a functional adverse effect."[68]

Imagine if tobacco promoters told us that yellow teeth are the only downside of smoking a pack of cigarettes per day.

In 2006, the National Research Council concluded, "It is apparent that fluorides have the ability to interfere with the functions of the brain and the body by direct and indirect means."[44] (See Appendix B.)

In 2017, a well-designed 12-year study funded by the US National Institutes of Health found a strong correlation between fluoride levels currently experienced by pregnant women in the US and lower IQ in their children at ages 4 & 6-12 years old. It was conducted largely by specialists in the field who had done similar studies on other environmental neurotoxins.[71]

> In 2018, they reported also that: "Higher *in utero* exposure to fluoride has an adverse impact on offspring cognitive development in the first three years of life."[71b]

Developmental Defects Increase with Fluoride Levels in Water
The IOM did not consider fluoride's adverse effects on the developing fetal GI tract or brain, despite the fact that defects in tooth enamel have been correlated with impaired brain development.

All enamel defects are indications of severe stress, because they result from systemic cellular disruption during prenatal and early postnatal life that can affect other ectodermally derived structures, including the brain. Chronologically distributed enamel defects are a valuable aid in neurological diagnosis, since they occur commonly in brain-damaged children.[72] Developmental enamel defects in primary teeth have been found at least twice as frequently in children with mental retardation as in children in a control group.[72b]

Some enamel defects are essentially birth defects resulting from a pregnant woman's consumption of fluoride. Similarly, a thin upper lip and flattened philtrum (the groove in the middle of the upper lip) are birth defects resulting from consumption of alcohol during pregnancy. They certainly signify more than a cosmetic effect, as does the grey-blue line on the gums of people with lead poisoning.

Dental studies show that the prevalence and severity of developmental defects of enamel in children increase significantly as fluoride levels in drinking water increase from less than 0.2 mg/l to more than 0.7 mg/l.[73-76] Fluoride supplements (0.25 to 0.75 mg/day) are also associated with developmental defects of enamel.[77] Fluoride levels in amniotic fluid have been positively correlated in a dose-response relationship with fluoride content and pathology of fetal bones – with significantly greater fluoride levels in fetuses born to mothers with dental fluorosis.[78]

As discussed in Chapter 1, prenatal fluoride is a risk factor for preterm birth, and infants born preterm are more frequently affected by tooth enamel defects, compared with infants born at term.[79]

Choi et al. (2015) found that developmental neurotoxicity was associated with dental fluorosis. Children with fluoride-induced mottling of their teeth – even the mildest form that appears as whitish specks on the enamel – showed lower performance on some neuropsychological tests.[80,81]

Genetic Susceptibility to Fluoride's Adverse Effects

Fluorosis severity does not depend just on the amount of fluoride one consumes. There are individual genetic and metabolic factors involved (as there are in ASD). Animal studies reveal a genetic component in the pathogenesis of dental fluorosis and in bone response to fluoride exposure.[82] In humans, severity of dental fluorosis varies individually at the same level of intake.[83]

Genetic sensitivity to fluoride's adverse neurological effects was confirmed by Zhang et al. (2015), who found that children with a variation of the COMT gene, which is associated with cognitive performance, had steeper cognitive decline from exposure to fluoride. Also, poor IQ scores were observed in the high fluoride exposure group (1.4 mg/l) compared with controls (0.63 mg/l).[84] Note: for generations, the recommended fluoride level in US drinking water was allowed to range up to 1.7 mg/l.

Fluorinated Pharmaceuticals in Pregnancy and Autism

In genetically susceptible individuals, autism may result from maternal exposure of a fetus to minute concentrations of pharmaceuticals, such as Prozac, a selective serotonin reuptake inhibitor (SSRI).[85] Because serotonin is critical to fetal brain development, concerns have arisen regarding prenatal exposure to SSRIs that manipulate serotonin levels.[86] Serotonin elevation in the blood is one of the better-documented and consistent findings in autism and is probably gastrointestinal in origin.[87] Note: 95% of the serotonin in the body is located in the gut.

Research shows that prenatal exposure to SSRIs is associated with an increased risk of autism.[88] A major study published in December 2015 looked at outcomes of 145,456 pregnancies over 12 years. The University of Montreal researchers found that taking SSRIs during the second or third trimester of pregnancy more than doubled a child's risk of being diagnosed with autism by age seven.[89]

Two of the most commonly prescribed SSRIs, Prozac (fluoxetine) and Paxil, contain fluorinated compounds. According to Gary M. Whitford, PhD, DMD, an expert on fluoride metabolism, a 20 mg dose of fluoxetine can provide up to 3.3 mg of fluoride, "depending on how much fluoride ion is released during the drug's metabolism."[90] Dr. Whitford was a key member of the Institute of Medicine panel that determined dietary reference intakes for fluoride.

SSRIs, Preeclampsia, and Autism
Taking SSRIs during pregnancy is also associated with preeclampsia, the dangerous pregnancy complication with immediate and life-long consequences for mother and child. In a study involving 5,731 pregnant women, the incidence of preeclampsia was 15.2% among those who continued SSRIs beyond the first trimester, compared to 2.4% among nonusers.[91]

Preeclampsia also increases the risk of having a child with ASD, and risk increases with greater preeclampsia severity.[92,93] As discussed in Chapter 2, preeclampsia has the same key subcellular mechanism of pathogenesis as dental and skeletal fluorosis, endoplasmic reticulum (ER) stress. In fluorosis, fluoride clearly causes the ER stress. In preeclampsia the cause is unknown.

Autism spectrum disorder is related to ER stress induced by mutations in the genes encoding synaptic cell adhesion molecules, and PSD-95 is involved.[94,95] As discussed above, fluoride decreases the expression level of PSD-95 in the brain.

Prenatal Fluoride, Preterm Birth, and Autism
As documented in Chapter 1, substantial laboratory and clinical evidence shows that maternal fluoride consumption is a risk factor for preterm birth, a leading cause of long-term neurological disabilities in children. Preterm birth is also significantly associated with autism. Large-scale population-based studies show that the prevalence of autism is 2 to 4 times higher in preterm children than in children born at full-term.[96,97]

The preterm gut experiences abnormal bacterial colonization with a decreased rate of diversification and altered microbiome composition. It also has an increased number of pathogenic bacteria. [12] Placentas collected after preterm births have significantly lower levels of bacteria that act a bit like natural versions of medications used to stop preterm contractions.[98]

A 2015 review by Aagaard et al. concluded, "The maternal oral, vaginal, and gut microbiome influence the risk of pregnancy outcomes that have profound impacts upon the health of the neonate and infant, including preterm birth, preeclampsia, gestational diabetes, and excessive gestational weight gain."[99]

Prenatal fluoride is also a significant risk factor for giving birth to low birthweight babies, who then have an increased risk of autism. Researchers at the University of Pennsylvania found that 5% of low birthweight children were diagnosed with autism, compared to 1% of the general population. (See page 12.)

Fluoridated Water: Hypothyroidism, Autism, and ADHD
In 2015, a major population-level study that analyzed data from 99% of England's 8,020 general medical practices showed a positive association between patients diagnosed with hypothyroidism and fluoride levels in their drinking water. High hypothyroidism prevalence was 30% more likely in practices located in areas with fluoride levels in drinking water in excess of 0.3 mg/l. Practices located in the West Midlands (a wholly fluoridated area) were nearly twice as likely to report high hypothyroidism prevalence in comparison to Greater Manchester (nonfluoridated area).[100]

The study did not include undiagnosed subclinical hypothyroidism. The National Research Council (2006) said that in pregnant women, subclinical hypothyroidism is associated with "decreased IQ of their offspring."[101] Klein et al. (2001) found an inverse correlation between severity of women's hypothyroidism and the IQ of their children.[102]

Fluoride's adverse effects on thyroid function are well documented. Thyroid hormones are essential for fetal and neonatal brain development. Even slight alterations during critical periods of development can have severe consequences on the development of the child.[103]

Andersen et al. (2015) observed that children born to mothers with thyroid dysfunction had an increased risk of developing autism spectrum disorder, attention-deficit/hyperactivity disorders (ADHD), and psychiatric disease in adolescence and young adulthood.[104]

The most common neurodevelopmental disorder of childhood is ADHD. Another large-scale population-based study in 2015 revealed that artificial water fluoridation prevalence was significantly positively associated with ADHD prevalence in the US. After controlling for socioeconomic status, each 1% increase in artificial fluoridation prevalence in 1992 was associated with approximately 67,000 to 131,000 additional ADHD diagnoses from 2003 to 2011.[105]

More Fluoride Absorbed from Artificially Fluoridated Water
Fluoridation promoters claim that because fluoride compounds have always been naturally present in drinking water, fluoride cannot be a factor in the increasing prevalence of developmental neurotoxicity. However, they overlook the fact that the degree of absorption of any fluoride compound after ingestion is correlated with its solubility.

The readily water-soluble industrial fluorides (sodium fluoride, sodium silicofluoride, fluorosilicic acid) used to artificially fluoridate drinking water are rapidly and almost completely absorbed, in contrast to low-soluble natural compounds such as calcium fluoride. The solubility of fluoride correlates generally with the degree of toxicity.[83,106]

Industrial fluorides are added to nearly three-fourths of US public water supplies; therefore substantial amounts of fluoride are also ingested from foods and beverages processed in fluoridated cities. Note: women are advised to drink more water when pregnant.

Fluoride, Copper, and Autism Spectrum Disorder
Water fluoridation chemicals have been shown to increase the leaching of lead and copper from brass plumbing fixtures into tap water.[107] (See Appendix C.) Copper has an antagonistic relationship with zinc. Excess copper levels and zinc deficiency are common in children diagnosed with an autism spectrum disorder.[108]

Due to the multifaceted effect of zinc on gut development, it is likely that insufficient zinc supply will affect development of the fetal GI tract, contributing to many of the reported GI problems associated with autism.[109]

Prenatal Fluoride: All Risk and No Benefit
The US Food and Drug Administration (FDA) classified fluoride as a Pregnancy Category C drug, which "may pose risks similar to a drug in Category X." The risks of a Category X drug clearly outweigh potential benefits.[110]

> **"Fluoride has no known essential function in human growth and development and no signs of fluoride deficiency have been identified."** – European Food Safety Authority.[111]

What are the potential benefits of ingesting fluoride during pregnancy? For the child, none. The FDA has long prohibited claims that prenatal fluoride supplements benefit children.[112] For the mother, the CDC said, "No published studies confirm the effectiveness of fluoride supplements in controlling dental caries among persons ages >16 years."[113] A 2015 Cochrane Review could not identify any evidence determining the effectiveness of water fluoridation for preventing caries in adults.[114] (Also see Appendix D.)

Lack of Fluoride-Pregnancy Research
As the National Scientific Council on the Developing Child points out: "There is no credible way to determine a safe level of exposure to a potentially toxic substance without explicit research that differentiates its impact on adults from the greater likelihood of its adverse influences on the developing brain during pregnancy."[62]

"The available studies of fluoride effects on human development are few and have some significant shortcomings," the National Research Council said in 2006 when it recommended: "Additional data from both the experimental and the clinical sciences are needed."[115]

A decade later, human research into prenatal fluoride and fetal brain development is conspicuously missing, despite the reality that US babies in the womb are needlessly exposed to the developmental neurotoxin fluoride, and that autism spectrum disorders are becoming epidemic. A PubMed Title/Abstract search for *autism* shows nearly 400 studies per month were published in the first half of 2018. For *fluoride*: 165 studies per month. For *autism* AND *fluoride*: only two new studies were published.

In the Saarland University study discussed above, when Loskill et al. exposed artificial teeth to a solution of 1,000 mg/l fluoride (the concentration in toothpaste) for five minutes, all bacteria species tested exhibited lower adhesion forces by a factor of two.

It is not known how lower concentrations and longer durations of fluoride exposure affect bacterial adhesion and colonization in the developing GI tract. However, when pregnant women daily used a mouthwash containing 225 mg/l of fluoride, even though they did not swallow it, colonization of their infants by bacteria was delayed by four months.[116]

Also, an extremely low concentration of fluoride in saliva is said to inhibit cariogenic bacteria – the *systemic* benefit that is the primary rationale for fluoridating America's drinking water. (See page 50.)

The gut–brain connection is attracting a lot of scientific research. A PubMed search for *gut brain* shows that about 75 new studies per month were published in the first half of 2018. In contrast, a search for *gut brain fluoride* yields zero results, ever.

Health of Maternal Microbiome Determines Autism Risk
In July 2018, researchers showed that a child's risk of developing autistic and other neurodevelopmental disorders is reduced when a pregnant woman has a healthy equilibrium of the diverse microorganisms in her gut. John Lukens, PhD, said it's really important to figure out how to modulate a mother's microbiome as "effectively and safely as we can," and that this can be easily done by modifying her diet.[117]

Again, fluoride was not considered, but as the research documented in this volume indicates: a common-sense strategy is to not swallow antibacterial substances. Don't drink fluoridated water.

Lukens also said a way to prevent autism is to block an inflammatory immune system molecule (IL-17a), but a pharmaceutical approach would be much more complex because of the risk of side effects.

Avoiding fluoride consumption can also reduce IL-17. Another 2018 study found that when rats were administered a human-equivalent dose of fluoride for 75 days, tissue inflammation and expression of IL-17 were significantly higher.[118] In mice chronically exposed to sodium fluoride, pathways related to IL-17 are over-expressed.[119]

Another July 2018 study found that reduced diversity and abundance of microorganisms in the gut microbiome of women is correlated with increased arterial stiffness. As discussed (page 34), fluoride exposure is linked to arterial stiffness and calcification, which lead to hypertension, a primary feature of preeclampsia.

We can no longer wait for the research community to come to the rescue. To better ensure the health of their children, mothers-to-be should avoid consumption of fluoride in tap water, bottled water, and beverages made in fluoridated cities – especially if they have dental fluorosis, the visible evidence of their genetic susceptibility to fluoride's systemic toxicity.

References – Prenatal Fluoride and Autism

1. Grandjean P, Landrigan PJ. Neurobehavioral effects of developmental toxicity. *Lancet Neurol.* 2014 Mar;13(3):330–338.

2. Choi AL, Sun GF, Zhang Y, Grandjean P. Developmental fluoride neurotoxicity: a systematic review and meta-analysis. *Environ Health Perspect.* 2012 Oct; 120(10):1362–1368.

3. Breaker RR. New insight on the response of bacteria to fluoride. *Caries Res.* 2012;46(1):78–81.

4. Loskill P, Zeitz C, Grandthyll S, et al. Reduced adhesion of oral bacteria on hydroxyapatite by fluoride treatment. *Langmuir.* 2013 May 7;29(18): 5528–5533.

5. Weiss J. After 50 years scientists gain clues how fluoride actually protects teeth. *Medical Daily.* May 1, 2013.

6. Dunne WM. Bacterial adhesion: seen any good biofilms lately? *Clin Microbiol Rev.* 2002 Apr;15(2):155–166.

7. Hao WL, Lee YK. Microflora of the gastrointestinal tract: a review. In: Spencer JFT, Spencer RD, eds. *Methods in Molecular Biology.* Vol. 268. *Public Health Microbiology: Methods and Protocols.* Humana Press. 2004.

8. Rodríguez JM, Murphy K, Stanton C, et al. The composition of the gut microbiota throughout life, with an emphasis on early life. *Microb Ecol Health Dis.* 2015 Feb 2;26:26050.

9. Sanz Y. Gut microbiota and probiotics in maternal and infant health. *Am J Clin Nutr.* 2011 Dec;94(6 Suppl):2000S–2005S.

10. Chu DM, Antony KM, Aagaard KM, et al. The early infant gut microbiome varies in association with a maternal high-fat diet. *Genome Med.* 2016 Aug 9;8(1):77.

11. Collado MC, Rautava S, Aakko J, Isolauri E, Salminen S. Human gut colonisation may be initiated *in utero* by distinct microbial communities in the placenta and amniotic fluid. *Sci Rep.* 2016 Mar 22;6:23129.

12. Rautava S. Early microbial contact, the breast milk microbiome and child health. *J Dev Orig Health Dis.* 2016 Feb;7(1):5–14.

13. Ardissone AN, de la Cruz DM, Davis-Richardson AG, et al. Meconium microbiome analysis identifies bacteria correlated with premature birth. *PLoS One.* 2014;9(3):e90784.

14. Cao B, Stout MJ, Lee I, Mysorekar IU. Placental microbiome and its role in preterm birth. *Neoreviews*. 2014 Dec 1;15(12):e537–e545.

15. Rautava S, Collado MC, Salminen S, Isolauri E. Probiotics modulate host-microbe interaction in the placenta and fetal gut: a randomized, double-blind, placebo-controlled trial. *Neonatology*. 2012;102(3):178–184.

16. Weng M, Walker WA. The role of gut microbiota in programming the immune phenotype. *J Dev Orig Health Dis*. 2013 Jun;4(3):203–214.

17. Chlubek D, Mokrzynski S, Machoy Z, Olszewska M. Fluorides in the body of the mother and in the fetus. III. Fluorides in amniotic fluid. *Ginekol Pol*. 1995 Nov;66(11):614–617.

18. Ron M, Singer L, Menczel J, Kidroni G. Fluoride concentration in amniotic fluid and fetal cord and maternal plasma. *Eur J Obstet Gynecol Reprod Biol*. 1986 Apr;21(4):213–218.

19. Brambilla E, Belluomo G, Malerba A, Buscaglia M, Strohmenger L. Oral administration of fluoride in pregnant women, and the relation between concentration in maternal plasma and in amniotic fluid. *Arch Oral Biol*. 1994 Nov;39(11):991–994.

20. Institute of Medicine. *Dietary Reference Intakes for Calcium, Phosphorus, Magnesium, Vitamin D, and Fluoride*. Washington, DC: National Academies Press; 1997:309.

21. Oliveby A, Twetman S, Ekstrand J. Diurnal fluoride concentration in whole saliva in children living in a high- and a low-fluoride area. *Caries Res*. 1990;24(1):44–47.

22. *Health Effects of Water Fluoridation: a Review of the Scientific Evidence*. A report on behalf of the Royal Society of New Zealand and the Office of the Prime Minister's Chief Science Advisor. August 2014.

23. Collado MC, Cernada M, Bauer C, Vento M, Perez-Martinez G. Microbial ecology and host-microbiota interactions during early life stages. *Gut Microbes*. 2012 July1;3(4):352–365.

24. Petrof EO, Claud EC, Gloor GB. Microbial ecosystems therapeutics: a new paradigm in medicine? *Benef Microbes*. 2013 Mar 1;4(1):53–65.

25. Finegold SM, Molitoris D, Song Y, et al. Gastrointestinal microflora studies in late-onset autism. *Clin Infect Dis*. 2002 Sep 1;35(Suppl 1):S6–S16.

26. Kang DW, Park JG, Krajmalnik-Brown R, et al. Reduced incidence of prevotella and other fermenters in intestinal microflora of autistic children. *PLoS One*. 2013 Jul 3;8(7):e68322.

27. Krajmalnik-Brown R, Lozupone C, Kang DW, Adams JB. Gut bacteria in children with autism spectrum disorders: challenges and promise of studying how a complex community influences a complex disease. *Microb Ecol Health Dis*. 2015 Mar 12;26:26914.

28. Sajdel-Sulkowska EM, Zabielski R. Gut microbiome and brain-gut axis in autism: aberrant development of gut-brain communication and reward circuitry. In: Fitzgerald M, ed. *Recent Advances in Autism Spectrum Disorders*. Vol. 1. Intech; 2013:61–79; 2013.

29. de Theije CG, Wopereis H, Ramadan M, et al. Altered gut microbiota and activity in a murine model of autism spectrum disorders. *Brain Behav Immun*. 2014 Mar;37:197–206.

30. Mazmanian SK, Liu CH, Tzianabos AO, Kasper DL. An immunomodulatory molecule of symbiotic bacteria directs maturation of the host immune system. *Cell*. 2005 Jul 15;122(1):107–118.

31. Hsiao EY, McBride SW, Hsien S, et al. The microbiota modulates gut physiology and behavioral abnormalities associated with autism. *Cell*. 2013 Dec 19;155(7):1451–1463.

   Potera C. Probiotic heals leaky guts in mice, improving autism-like symptoms. *Microbe*. April 2014.

32. Petra AI, Panagiotidou S, Hatziagelaki E, Stewart JM, Conti P, Theoharides TC. Gut-microbiota-brain axis and its effect on neuropsychiatric disorders with suspected immune dysregulation. *Clin Ther*. 2015 May 1;37 (5):984–995.

33. Furness JB, Kunze WA, Clerc N. Nutrient tasting and signaling mechanisms in the gut. II. The intestine as a sensory organ: neural, endocrine and immune responses. *Am J Physiol*. 1999 Nov;277(5 Pt 1):G922–928.

34. Lee YK, Mazmanian SK. Has the microbiota played a critical role in the evolution of the adaptive immune system? *Science*. 2010 Dec 24; 330(6012): 1768–1773.

35. Round JL, Mazmanian SK. The gut microbiota shapes intestinal immune responses during health and disease. *Nat Rev Immunol*. 2009 May;9(5):313–323.

36. Isolauri E, Rautava S, Kalliomäki M, Kirjavainen P, Salminen S. Role of probiotics in food hypersensitivity. *Curr Opin Allergy Clin Immunol*. 2002 Jun;2(3):263–271.

37. Pessah IN, Seegal RF, Lein PJ, et al. Immunologic and neurodevelopmental susceptibilities of autism. *Neurotoxicology*. 2008 May; 29(3):531–544.

38. Ochoa-Repáraz J, Mielcarz DW, Ditrio LE, et al. Central nervous system demyelinating disease protection by the human commensal Bacteroides fragilis depends on polysaccharide A expression. *J Immunol.* 2010 Oct 1; 185(7):4101–4108.

39. Hardan AY, Fung LK, Frazier T, et al. A proton spectroscopy study of white matter in children with autism. *Prog Neuropsychopharmacol Biol Psychiatry.* 2015 Nov 16;66:48–53.

40. Wei H, Ma Y, Liu J, Ding C, Hu F, Yu L. Proteomic analysis of cortical brain tissue from the BTBR mouse model of autism: evidence for changes in STOP and myelin-related proteins. *Neuroscience.* 2015 Nov 10;312:26–34.

41. Shimura N, Onisi M. The effect of NaF on the bacterial production of polysaccharide and subsequent adsorption on hydroxyapatite. *J Dent Res.* 1978 Sep-Oct;57(9-10):928–931.

42. Luengpailin S, Banas JA, Doyle RJ. Modulation of glucan-binding protein activity in streptococci by fluoride. *Biochim Biophys Acta.* 2000 May 1;1474(3):346–352.

43. Vetvicka V, Vannucci L, Sima P. Role of B-glucan in biology of gastrointestinal tract. *J Nat Sci.* 2015 Jul;1(7):e129.

44. National Research Council. *Fluoride in drinking water: A scientific review of EPA's standards.* Washington, DC: National Academies Press; 2006. Page 222.

45. Connett M. Fluoride's effect on the fetal brain. Fluoride Action Network. April 2015.

   National Research Council. Op cit., 91.

46. Stoner R, Chow ML, Boyle MP, et al. Patches of disorganization in the neocortex of children with autism. *N Engl J Med.* 2014 Mar 27;370(13): 1209–1219.

47. Lahiri DK, Sokol DK, Erickson C, Ray B, Ho CY, Maloney B. Autism as early neurodevelopmental disorder: evidence for an sAPPα-mediated anabolic pathway. *Front Cell Neurosci.* 2013 Jun 21;7:94.

48. Kameno Y, Iwata K, Matsuzaki H, et al. Serum levels of soluble platelet endothelial cell adhesion molecule-1 and vascular cell adhesion molecule-1 are decreased in subjects with autism spectrum disorder. *Mol Autism.* 2013 Jun 17;4(1):19.

49. Plioplys AV, Hemmens SE, Regan CM. Expression of a neural cell adhesion molecule serum fragment is depressed in autism. *J Neuropsychiatry Clin Neurosci.* 1990 Fall;2(4):413–417.

50. Betancur C, Sakurai T, Buxbaum JD. The emerging role of synaptic cell-adhesion pathways in the pathogenesis of autism spectrum disorders. *Trends Neurosci.* 2009 Jul;32(7):402–412.

51. Sakurai T. The role of NrCAM in neural development and disorders: beyond a simple glue in the brain. *Mol Cell Neurosci.* 2012 Mar;49(3): 351–363.

52. Xia T, Zhang M, He WH, He P, Wang AG. Effects of fluoride on neural cell adhesion molecules mRNA and protein expression levels in primary rat hippocampal neurons. *Zhonghua Yu Fang Yi Xue Za Zhi.* 2007 Nov;41(6): 475–478.

53. Zhang M, Wang AG, He WH, et al. Effects of fluoride on the expression of NCAM, oxidative stress, and apoptosis in primary cultured hippocampal neurons. *Toxicology.* 2007 Jul 17;236(3):208–216.

54. Beggs HE, Baragona SC, Hemperly JJ, Maness PF. NCAM140 interacts with the focal adhesion kinase p125(fak) and the SRC-related tyrosine kinase p59(fyn). *J Biol Chem.* 1997 Mar 28;272(13):8310–8319.

55. Zielinska E. Building and breaking synapses. Thomas Jefferson University press release. October 19, 2015.

56. Wang SQ, Fang F, Xue ZG, Cang J, Zhang XG. Neonatal sevoflurane anesthesia induces long-term memory impairment and decreases hippocampal PSD-95 expression without neuronal loss. *Eur Rev Med Pharmacol Sci.* 2013 Apr;17(7):941–950.

57. Qian W, Miao K, Li T, Zhang Z. Effect of selenium on fluoride-induced changes in synaptic plasticity in rat hippocampus. *Biol Trace Elem Res.* 2013 Nov;155(2):253–260.

58. Zhu W, Zhang J, Zhang Z. Effects of fluoride on synaptic membrane fluidity and PSD-95 expression level in rat hippocampus. *Biol Trace Elem Res.* 2011 Feb;139(2):197–203.

59. Goldberg ME, Cantillo J, Larijani GE, Torjman M, Vekeman D, Schieren H. Sevoflurane versus isoflurane for maintenance of anesthesia: are serum inorganic fluoride ion concentrations of concern? *Anesth Analg.* 1996 Jun;82 (6):1268–1272.

60. Mundy W, Padilla S, Shafer T, et al. Building a database of developmental neurotoxicants: Evidence from human and animal studies. Neurotoxicology Division. US EPA. 2009.

61. Mundy WR, Padilla S, Breier JM, et al. Expanding the test set: Chemicals with potential to disrupt mammalian brain development. *Neurotoxicol Teratol.* 2015 Nov-Dec;52(Pt A):25–35.

61b. Carter CJ, Blizard RA. Autism genes are selectively targeted by environmental pollutants including pesticides, heavy metals, bisphenol A, phthalates and many others in food, cosmetics or household products. *Neurochemistry International*. 2016 Dec. Vol 101. Pages 83–109.

62. National Scientific Council on the Developing Child. *Early exposure to toxic substances damages brain architecture: Working Paper No. 4*. 2006.

63. Shimonovitz S, Patz D, Ever-Hadani P, et al. Umbilical cord fluoride serum levels may not reflect fetal fluoride status. *J Perinat Med*. 1995;23(4): 279–782.

64. Burd L, Blair J, Dropps K. Prenatal alcohol exposure, blood alcohol concentrations and alcohol elimination rates for the mother, fetus and newborn. *J. Perinatal*. (2012) 32, 652–659.

65. Brien JF, Loomis CW, Tranmer J, McGrath M. Disposition of ethanol in human maternal venous blood and amniotic fluid. *Am J Obstet Gynecol*. 1983 May 15;146(2):181–186.

66. Institute of Medicine. Op cit., 309.

67. Ibid., 60.

68. Institute of Medicine (2000). *DRI Dietary Reference Intakes: Applications in Dietary Assessment*. Using the Tolerable Upper Intake Level for Nutrient Assessment of Groups. Frequently Asked Questions; Table 6-1.

69. Ibid., 315.

70. Ibid., 52.

71. Bashash M, Thomas D, Hu H, et al. Prenatal fluoride exposure and cognitive outcomes in children at 4 and 6-12 years of age in Mexico. *Environ Health Perspect*. 2017 Sep 19;125(9):097017.

71b. OP V–2 Prenatal fluoride exposure and neurobehavior among children 1–3 years of age in Mexico. Conference Paper in *Occupational and Environmental Medicine* 75(Suppl 1):A10.1-A10. March 2018.

72. Aminabadi NA, Oskouei SG, Pouralibaba F, Jamali Z, Pakdel F. Enamel defects of human primary dentition as virtual memory of early developmental events. *J Dent Res Dent Clin Dent Prospects*. 2009 Autumn;3(4):110–116.

72b. Bhat M, Nelson KB. Developmental enamel defects in primary teeth in children with cerebral palsy, mental retardation, or hearing defects: a review. *Adv Dent Res*. 1989 Sep;3(2):132–142.

73. Ekanayake L, van der Hoek W. Dental caries and developmental defects of enamel in relation to fluoride levels in drinking water in an arid area of Sri Lanka. *Caries Res*. 2002 Nov-Dec;36(6):398–404.

74. Nunn JH, Rugg-Gunn AJ, Ekanayake L, Saparamadu KD. Prevalence of developmental defects of enamel in areas with differing water fluoride levels and socio-economic groups in Sri Lanka and England. *Int Dent J*. 1994 Apr; 44(2):165–173.

75. Weeks KJ, Milsom KM, Lennon MA. Enamel defects in 4- to 5-year-old children in fluoridated and nonfluoridated parts of Cheshire, UK. *Caries Res*. 1993;27(4):317–320.

76. Wong HM, McGrath C, Lo EC, King NM. Association between developmental defects of enamel and different concentrations of fluoride in the public water supply. *Caries Res*. 2006;40(6):481–486.

77. Hiller KA, Wilfart G, Schmalz G. Developmental enamel defects in children with different fluoride supplementation – a follow-up study. *Caries Res*. 1998;32(6):405–411.

78. Shi J, Dai G, Zhang Z. Relationship between bone fluoride content, pathological change in bone of aborted fetuses and maternal fluoride level. *Zhonghua Yu Fang Yi Xue Za Zhi*. 1995 Mar;29(2):103–105.

79. Hall RK. Prevalence of developmental defects of tooth enamel (DDE) in a pediatric hospital department of dentistry population (1). *Adv Dent Re*s. 1989 Sep;3(2):114–119.

80. Choi AL, Zhang Y, Sun G, et al. Association of lifetime exposure to fluoride and cognitive functions in Chinese children: a pilot study. *Neurotoxicol Teratol*. 2015 Jan-Feb;47:96–101.

81. Grandjean P. Mottled fluoride debate. *Chemical Brain Drain*. December 17, 2014.

82. Everett ET. Fluoride's effects on the formation of teeth and bones, and the influence of genetics. *J Dent Res*. 2011 May;90(5):552–560.

83. European Food Safety Authority. Scientific Opinion on Dietary Reference Values for Fluoride. *EFSA J*. 2013;11(8):3332. Page 11.

84. Zhang S, Zhang X, Liu H, et al. Modifying effect of COMT gene polymorphism and a predictive role for proteomics analysis in children's intelligence in endemic fluorosis area in Tianjin, China. *Toxicol Sci*. 2015 Apr;144(2):238–245.

85. Kaushik G, Thomas MA, Aho KA. Psychoactive pharmaceuticals as environmental contaminants may disrupt highly inter-connected nodes in an Autism-associated protein-protein interaction network. *BMC Bioinformatics.* 2015;16 Suppl 7:S3.

86. Harrington RA, Lee LC, Crum RM, Zimmerman AW, Hertz-Picciotto I. Serotonin hypothesis of autism: implications for selective serotonin reuptake inhibitor use during pregnancy. *Autism Res.* 2013 Jun;6(3):149–168.

87. McGinnis WR, Audhya T, Edelson SM. Proposed toxic and hypoxic impairment of a brainstem locus in autism. *Int J Environ Res Public Health.* 2013 Dec; 10(12):6955-7000.

88. Kupelian D. Top Doc: media bias on antidepressants 'astounding.' Repeated studies show SSRI use during pregnancy linked to autism, but press AWOL. WND. August 1, 2014.

89. Raillant-Clark W. Taking antidepressants during pregnancy increases risk of autism by 87 percent. Université de Montréal. December 14, 2005.

Boukhris T, Sheehy O, Mottron L, Bérard A. Antidepressant use during pregnancy and the risk of autism spectrum disorder in children. *JAMA Pediatrics.* 2015 Dec 14:1–8.

90. Whyte MP, Totty WG, Lim VT, Whitford GM. Skeletal fluorosis from instant tea. *J Bone Miner Res.* 2008 May;23(5):759–769.

91. Toh S, Mitchell AA, Louik C, Werler MM, Chambers CD, Hernández-Díaz S. Selective serotonin reuptake inhibitor use and risk of gestational hypertension. *Am J Psychiatry.* 2009 Mar; 166(3):320–328.

92. Mann JR, McDermott S, Bao H, Hardin J, Gregg A. Pre-eclampsia, birth weight, and autism spectrum disorders. *J Autism Dev Disord.* 2010 May;40(5):548–554.

93. Walker CK, Krakowiak P, Baker A, Hansen RL, Ozonoff S, Hertz-Picciotto I. Preeclampsia, placental insufficiency, and autism spectrum disorder or developmental delay. *JAMA Pediatr.* 2015 Feb;169(2):154–162.

94. Fujita E, Dai H, Tanabe Y, et al. Autism spectrum disorder is related to endoplasmic reticulum stress induced by mutations in the synaptic cell adhesion molecule, CADM1. *Cell Death Dis.* 2010 Jun;1(6):e47.

95. Fujita-Jimbo E, Tanabe Y, Yu Z, et al. The association of GPR85 with PSD-95-neuroligin complex and autism spectrum disorder: a molecular analysis. *Mol Autism.* 2015;6:17.

96. Hwang YS, Weng SF, Cho CY, Tsai WH. Higher prevalence of autism in Taiwanese children born prematurely: a nationwide population-based study. *Res Dev Disabil.* 2013 Sep;34(9):2462–2468.

97. Singh GK, Kenney MK, Ghandour RM, Kogan MD, Lu MC. Mental health outcomes in US children and adolescents born prematurely or with low birthweight. *Depress Res Treat*. 2013;2013:570743.

98. Aagaard K, Ma J, Antony KM, Ganu R, Petrosino J, Versalovic J. The placenta harbors a unique microbiome. *Sci Transl Med*. 2014;6(237): 237ra265.

   Neergaard L. Bacteria live even in healthy placentas. WTOP. 5/24/2014.

99. Dunlop AL, Mulle JG, Ferranti EP, Edwards S, Dunn AB, Corwin EJ. Maternal microbiome and pregnancy outcomes that impact infant health: a review. *Adv Neonatal Care*. 2015 Dec;15(6):377–385.

100. Peckham S, Lowery D, Spencer S. Are fluoride levels in drinking water associated with hypothyroidism prevalence in England? A large observational study of GP practice data and fluoride levels in drinking water. *J Epidemiol Community Health*. 2015;0:1- 6.

101. National Research Council. Op cit., 236.

102. Klein RZ, Sargent JD, Larsen PR, Waisbren SE, Haddow JE, Mitchell ML. Relation of severity of maternal hypothyroidism to cognitive development of offspring. *J Med Screen*. 2001;8:18–20.

103. Parents of Fluoride-Poisoned Children (PFPC). Fluoride and Developmental Neurotoxicity. Comments submitted to the National Toxicology Program Board of Scientific Counselors. January 8, 2016.

104. Andersen SL, Olsen J, Laurberg P. Fetal programming by maternal thyroid disease. *Clin Endocrinol (Oxf)*. 2015;83(6):751–758.

105. Malin AJ, Till C. Exposure to fluoridated water and attention deficit hyperactivity disorder prevalence among children and adolescents in the United States: an ecological association. *Environ Health*. 2015;14:17.

106. Sauerheber R. Physiologic conditions affect toxicity of ingested industrial fluoride. *J Environ Public Health*. 2013;2013:439490.

   Overview of Fluoride Poisoning: Etiology and Pathogenesis. *Merck Manual*. December 2013.

107. MacArthur JD. Overdosed: fluoride, copper, and Alzheimer's disease. *Townsend Lett*. 2013;363:63–70. PregnancyAndFluorideDoNotMix.com/ author/FluorideCopperAlzheimersMacArthurOct2013.pdf

108. Bjorklund G. The role of zinc and copper in autism spectrum disorders. *Acta Neurobiol Exp (Wars)*. 2013;73(2):225–236.

109. Vela G, Stark P, Socha M, Sauer AK, Hagmeyer S, Grabrucker AM. Zinc in gut-brain interaction in autism and neurological disorders. *Neural Plast*. 2015;2015:972791.

110. US Food and Drug Administration. Summary of proposed rule on pregnancy and lactation labeling. *Federal Register*. 2008 May29;73(104): 30833-34.

111. European Food Safety Authority. Op cit., 2.

112. Institute of Medicine. Op cit., 304.

113. US Centers for Disease Control and Prevention. Recommendations for using fluoride to prevent and control dental caries in the United States. *Morb Mortal Rep*. August 17, 2001;50(14);3. Table 4 (footnote).

114. Iheozor-Ejiofor Z, Worthington HV, Walsh T, et al. Water fluoridation for the prevention of dental caries. *Cochrane Database Syst Rev*. 2015;6. Art. No.: CD010856.

115. National Research Council. Op cit., 203, 222.

116. Brambilla E, Felloni A, Gagliani M, Malerba A, García-Godoy F, Strohmenger L. Caries prevention during pregnancy: results of a 30-month study. *J Am Dent Assoc*. 1998 Jul;129(7):871–877.

117. Barney J. Autism risk determined by health of mom's gut, UVA research reveals. University of Virginia Health System press release. July 18, 2018.

   Lammert CR, Frost EL, Lukens JR, et al. Cutting edge: Critical roles for microbiota-mediated regulation of the immune system in a prenatal immune activation model of autism. *J Immunol*. 2018 Aug 1;201(3):845–850.

118. Quadri JA, Sarwar S, Shariff A, et al. Fluoride induced tissue hypercalcemia, IL-17 mediated inflammation and apoptosis lead to cardiomyopathy: Ultrastructural and biochemical findings. *Toxicology*. 2018 May 22;406-407:44–57.

119. Huo M, Han H, Sun Z, et al. Role of IL-17 pathways in immune privilege: A RNA deep sequencing analysis of the mice testis exposure to fluoride. *Sci Rep*. 2016 Aug 30;6:32173.

Afterwards

Infancy and Fluoride Do Not Mix

The amount of fluoride that breast-fed infants receive from their mother's milk is extremely low. It averages about 1 microgram (0.3–1.6 μg) of fluoride per kilogram of body weight per day.[1] Even when a mother's fluoride intake is high, fluoride levels in her breast milk remain at this very low level[2] – just as it does with lead, another EPA-designated *developmental neurotoxicant*. (See pages 53-54.)

> Breast milk does more than protect newborn infants from fluoride intake. It allows them to excrete the fluoride accumulated while in the womb. "Exclusively breast-fed infants not receiving a fluoride supplement showed negative fluoride balances up to the age of four months and excreted more fluoride than they ingested."[1]

For formula-fed infants, their fluoride intake depends on the concentration of fluoride in the water used to prepare their formula. "Use of water with 1.0 mg fluoride/liter compared to 0.15 mg/l increases the fluoride intake of the infant five-fold."[1]

The Iowa Fluoride Study found that "fluoride intake per day was highest from zero to three months: 0.075 mg/kg body weight" – 75 times the amount of fluoride consumed by a breast-fed infant. For most children, fluoridated water was the predominant source of fluoride.[1]

In nonfluoridated areas, parents are advised to feed their 6-month-old infant an unapproved drug containing 250 micrograms of fluoride – a daily dose 30 times the amount of fluoride that a 6-month-old (8 kg) breast-fed infant consumes.

> Children also swallow fluoride in toothpaste. Ingestion has been reported to be as high as 48% in young children 2 to 3 years old.[3] Worse, after dentists apply high-concentration fluoride gels and varnishes containing 12,300–22,500 ppm of fluoride to children's teeth, from 2–30 mg of fluoride may be swallowed.[4]

Fluoride has strong antimicrobial properties. When swallowed, fluoride may impair a newborn's developing immune system, because the GI tract is the primary site of interaction between microorganisms and the immune system. (See pages 49-51.)

Fluoridated Water and Life Decay

Fluoridation is claimed necessary because fluoridated kids have about 20% less tooth decay: measured by the number of decayed, missing, and filled teeth or tooth surfaces (present & past decay). But fluoride affects the entire body. So then what about fluoridated water's correlation with decayed and missing *years:* with disease and death?

Decayed Years: Fluoridation and Disease

Death rates from leading diseases average 2–26% higher in the most fluoridated states compared to the least fluoridated.[5,6]

Decayed Years	Average age-adjusted death rate per 100,000 pop.	Average age-adjusted death rate per 100,000 pop.	
Leading Causes of Death (2013)	30 states **<80%** fluoridated (avg. 58% • 2012)	20 states **>80%** fluoridated (avg. 93% • 2012)	% higher death rate in 20 most fluoridated states
Heart Disease (#1)	166.5	170.5	2.4%
Cancer (#2)	161.8	169.8	4.9%
Stroke (#5)	36.2	37.6	3.9%
Alzheimer's (#6)	23.5	25.6	8.9%
Diabetes (#7)	21.2	21.9	3.3%
Kidney Disease (#9)	12.7	14.4	13.4%

Decayed Years	Average age-adjusted death rate per 100,000 pop.	Average age-adjusted death rate per 100,000 pop.	
Leading Causes of Death (2013)	**10 least** fluoridated states (avg. 35% • 2012)	**10 most** fluoridated states (avg. 97% • 2012)	% higher death rate in 10 most fluoridated states
Heart Disease (#1)	157.0	167.2	6.5%
Cancer (#2)	156.0	167.9	7.6%
Stroke (#5)	36.3	38.5	6.1%
Alzheimer's (#6)	21.1	26.4	25.1%
Diabetes (#7)	20.7	21.7	4.8%
Kidney Dis. (#9)	11.8	14.9	26.3%

Missing Years: Fluoridation and Life Expectancy

The life expectancy of people living in the least fluoridated states averages 0.6 years longer than those in the most fluoridated states. Based on a highest national life expectancy of 84 years, that means people living in the most fluoridated states average about 12% more missing years than those in the least fluoridated states.[6,7]

Missing Years (2010)	28 states <80% fluoridated (avg. (55% • 2010)	22 states ≥80% fluoridated (91% • 2010)	% more missing years in 22 most fluoridated states
# of years below 84 years of life expectancy	5.1	5.7	11.8%

Fluoridation and Infant Mortality

Infant and neonatal death rates average 9–19% higher in the most fluoridated states compared to the least fluoridated.[5,6]

Infant Deaths per 1,000 live births for all races (2013)	10 least fluoridated states (avg. 35% • 2012)	10 most fluoridated states (avg. 97% • 2012)	% higher death rate in 10 most fluoridated states
Neonatal Deaths (under 28 days old)	3.6	4.3	19.4%
Infant Deaths (under 1 year old)	5.7	6.4	12.3%

The #2 leading cause of infant death:
"Disorders related to short gestation and low birthweight."

Infant Deaths /1,000 live births for all races (2013)	30 states <80% fluoridated (avg. 58% • 2012)	20 states >80% fluoridated (avg. 93% • 2012)	% higher death rate in 20 most fluoridated states
Neonatal Deaths (under 28 days old)	3.9	4.3	10.3%
Infant Deaths (under 1 year old)	5.9	6.4	8.5%

Fluoridated water's multiple correlations with life decay make a far more compelling case to stop fluoridation, than its single correlation with tooth decay did to start it in 1945 – based on dental survey data from the 1930s that has since been debunked.[8]

Correlation should be a wake-up call to investigate causation. For decades, however, research institutions in fluoridated nations have failed to challenge fluoridation "science," despite that it's long been known that fluoride increases inflammation and oxidative stress, cellular processes fundamental to the development of most diseases.

The Elephant in the Tomb

Ignoring fluoride exposure is especially irrational now, because new understandings of mechanisms common to age-related diseases often involve fluoride. A prime example is <u>endothelial cell dysfunction</u>. These crucial cells line the inside of blood vessels and form a selective blood-tissue barrier that protects every organ system in the body – and in the brain via the blood-brain barrier.

A major cause of vascular dementia is small vessel disease (SVD), which also triples the risk of stroke and contributes to Alzheimer's disease. A study published in July 2018 shows that endothelial cell dysfunction in the blood-brain barrier is the first pathological change in the development of SVD in older people.[9]

A study cited found that after exposure to the general anesthetic Sevoflurane, the blood-brain barrier is compromised due to "flattening of endothelial cell surfaces."[10]

Sevoflurane significantly increases blood fluoride levels (see page 53) and is associated with high rates of post-operative delirium, a common and often fatal disorder affecting as many as 50% of older people during surgery or hospitalization. The severity of post-operative delirium correlates directly to the severity of later cognitive impairment and decline.[11]

Another drug that increases blood fluoride levels is 5-fluorouracil, which in 2017 was found to "cause endothelial cell senescence and dysfunction."[12,13]

> In 2001, it was "demonstrated that sodium fluoride
> causes dramatic endothelial cell barrier dysfunction."[14]

In July 2018, researchers at the University of Exeter showed that key aspects of human cell aging can be reversed by decreasing levels of endothelial cells that are senescent (older cells that stop dividing). Professor Lorna Harries says a common mechanism in age-related diseases like dementia, cancer, and diabetes is the accumulation of these dysfunctional endothelial cells that are not just an effect of aging. "It's a reason why we age."[15]

An August 2018 study found a strong association between cellular senescence in the brain and the presence of tau-containing neurofibrillary tangles, whose accumulation is the most common pathology among degenerative brain diseases. Clearing even a small percentage of the senescent cells improves health span and delays age-associated diseases.[16]

Endothelial cell dysfunction is also a central mechanism in the pathophysiology of preeclampsia.[17] A marker of endothelial dysfunction is soluble Endoglin (sEng), whose levels are elevated in preeclampsia. Amniotic tissue cultures treated with sodium fluoride have significantly higher expression levels of sEng.[18]

A measure of endothelial dysfunction is arterial stiffness. A study published in May 2018 found that reduced cognitive performance in older people is independently associated with aortic stiffness.[19]

As discussed in Fluoride: Hypertension, Arterial Stiffness, and Preeclampsia (page 34), fluoride increases arterial calcification and stiffening that lead to hypertension. In people with fluorosis, the elastic properties of the ascending aorta are impaired.[20]

"Vascular Aging and Arterial Stiffness," a 2017 study, found that the "biological aging process is always associated with arterial stiffness, which is accelerated by arterial hypertension." Worldwide, it's estimated that 9.4 million deaths per year are related to arterial hypertension, a highly relevant risk factor for stroke, coronary artery disease, and heart failure.[21]

References – Afterword

1. European Food Safety Authority. Scientific Opinion on Dietary Reference Values for Fluoride. *EFSA J*. 2013;11(8):3332.

2. Institute of Medicine. *Dietary Reference Intakes for Calcium, Phosphorus, Magnesium, Vitamin D, and Fluoride*. National Academies Press; 1997:305.

3. Critical review of any new evidence on the hazard profile, health effects, and human exposure to fluoride and the fluoridating agents of drinking water. European Union. SCHER. 16 May 2011:21.

4. Lecompte EJ. Clinical application of topical fluoride products-risks, benefits and recommendations. *J Dent Res*. 1987 May;66(5):1066–71.

5. Xu J, Murphy SL, Kochanek KD, Bastian BA. Deaths: Final Data for 2013. *Natl Vital Stat Rep*. 2016 Feb 16;64(2):86–89, 98.

6. Percentage of state populations on community water systems receiving fluoridated water (2012 and 2010). National Water Fluoridation Statistics.

7. Measure of America 2013-2014. American Human Development Index by State. 2010. Page 45. Life Expectancy at Birth.

8. Ziegelbecker R. Fluoridated water and teeth. *Fluoride* 1981;14(3):123–28; Bryson C. *The Fluoride Deception*. Seven Stories Press;2004:43.

9. Barney J. Stabilizing endothelial cells could help tackle vascular dementia. American Association for the Advancement of Science. July 2018.

10. Acharya NK, Goldwaser EL, Forsberg MM, et al. Sevoflurane and isoflurane induce structural changes in brain vascular endothelial cells and increase blood-brain barrier permeability: Possible link to postoperative delirium and cognitive decline. *Brain Res*. 2015 Sep 16;1620:29–41.

11. Howe C. Severity of post-operative delirium relates to severity of cognitive decline. Hebrew SeniorLife Institute for Aging Research. 11/28/17.

12. Hull WE, Port RE, Herrmann R, et al. Metabolites of 5-fluorouracil in plasma and urine... *Cancer Res*. 1988 Mar 15;48(6):1680–1688.

13. Altieri P, Murialdo R, Barisione C, et al. 5-fluorouracil causes endothelial cell senescence... *Br J Pharmacol.* 2017 Nov;174(21):3713–3726.

14. Wang P, Verin AD, Birukova A, et al. Mechanisms of sodium fluoride-induced endothelial cell barrier dysfunction: role of MLC phosphorylation. *Am J Physiol Lung Cell Mol Physiol*. 2001 Dec;281(6):L1472–1483.

15. Key aspects of human cell aging reversed by new compounds. University of Exeter. August 7, 2018.

16. Musi N, Valentine JM, Sickora KR, et al. Tau protein aggregation is associated with cellular senescence in the brain. *Aging Cell*. 2018 Aug 20:e12840.h

17. Meeme A, Buga GA, Mammen M, Namugowa A. Endothelial dysfunction and arterial stiffness in pre-eclampsia demonstrated by the EndoPAT method. *Cardiovasc J Afr*. 2017 Jan/Feb 23;28(1):23-29.

18. Tskitishvili E, Sharentuya N, Temma-Asano K, et al. Oxidative stress-induced S100B protein from placenta and amnion affects soluble endoglin release from endothelial cells. *Mol Hum Reprod*. 2010;16(3):188–199. Figures 5C, 5D.

19. Kennedy G, Meyer D, Hardman RJ, et al. Physical fitness and aortic stiffness explain the reduced cognitive performance associated with increasing age in older people. *J Alzheimers Dis*. 2018;63(4):1307-1316.

20. Varol E, Akcay S, Ersoy IH, et al. Aortic elasticity is impaired in patients with endemic fluorosis. *Biol Trace Elem Res*. 2010 Feb;133(2):121-127.

21. Mikael LR, Paiva AMG, Gomes MM, et al. Vascular aging and arterial stiffness. *Arq Bras Cardiol*. 2017 Sep;109(3):253-258.

Appendices

Appendix A

Unborn Babies are Overexposed to Fluoride in Tap Water

The *Adequate Intake Level* of fluoride that health authorities say women, including pregnant women, should consume daily is 3 mg of fluoride. Most of that intake is from drinking fluoridated tap water.[1] "Intake Levels" are measured in milligrams of fluoride per kilogram of body weight. Safety thresholds are based on intake level per day.

Tolerable Upper Intake Level of Fluoride
In 1997, the US Institute of Medicine (IOM) established 0.10 mg/kg per day as the *Tolerable Upper Intake Level* (UL) of fluoride for children under 9 years old.[2]

A fetal fluoride UL was not determined. But now it must be, because since then a team of researchers at EPA's Neurotoxicology Division is finding "substantial evidence" that fluoride is a "developmental neurotoxicant" (like lead and alcohol). Also because, the fluoride UL is based on a gross biomarker: defects in developing teeth, not in the developing brain. (See pages 53-56.)

The IOM said a fetal UL would be "significantly lower" because in the unborn fetus, "sensitivity increases due to active placental transfer, accumulation of certain nutrients in the amniotic fluid, and rapid development of the brain."[2] A fetal fluoride UL "significantly lower" than the 0.10 mg/kg/day for children would reasonably be at least a fifth of that – 0.02 mg/kg/day – a level that is comparable to the fluoride intake babies in the womb receive when their mothers drink fluoridated water throughout the day, as they're advised to do.[3]

Eight cups of US tap water optimally fluoridated at 0.7 mg/l contain 1.33 mg of fluoride. About 85% of the ingested fluoride is absorbed,[4] so 1.13 mg enters the bloodstream. Late in the third trimester, a 3 kg baby weighs about 5% of his mother's weight (60 kg). If fluoride is evenly distributed, then the baby in the womb takes in 5% of 1.13 mg = 0.056 mg of fluoride. **The fetal fluoride intake level (0.056 ÷ 3) is about 0.02 mg/kg**. This suggests that in communities where tap water is fluoridated, babies in the womb are being exposed to fluoride at their Tolerable Upper Intake Level.

> *"A population mean intake at the UL suggests that as much as half of the population is consuming levels above the UL.* ***This would represent a very serious population risk of adverse effects.*** *"* – Institute of Medicine (2000)[5]

Fluoride Toothpaste Warning

Another safety threshold is the 1997 FDA-mandated warning for fluoride toothpaste that advises parents to: "Get medical help or contact a Poison Control Center right away" if their child accidentally swallows more toothpaste than is used for brushing.[6] For 3-6 year olds, that amount is only a *pea-sized dab* of toothpaste that contains 0.25 mg of fluoride.[7]

If a 20 kg 5-year-old child swallows that much toothpaste, he absorbs about 0.20 mg of fluoride, so his *one-time* fluoride intake level $(0.20 \div 20) = 0.01$ mg/kg. This is comparable to a 3rd-trimester baby's with every 4 cups of fluoridated water its mother drinks.

Worse: that unborn child's fluoride intake level is *daily* during the crucial months when its brain has a "heightened susceptibility... to developmental disruption."[8]

> Note: It is unlikely that ingested fluoride is evenly distributed. Animal research has found fluoride concentrations four times higher in the pineal gland than in the skull or the brain.[9]

References

1. National Research Council (2006). *Fluoride in drinking water: A scientific review of EPA's standards*. Appendix B. Measures of Exposure to Fluoride in the United States: Tables B-17 and B-10.

2. Institute of Medicine (1997). *Dietary Reference Intakes for Calcium, Phosphorus, Magnesium, Vitamin D, and Fluoride*.

3. Tips for Good Oral Health During Pregnancy. From *Oral Health Care During Pregnancy: A National Consensus Statement*. 2012. Funded by HHS.

4. European Food Safety Authority. Scientific Opinion on Dietary Reference Values for Fluoride. *EFSA J*. 2013;11(8):3332. Page 12.

5. Institute of Medicine (2000). *DRI Dietary Reference Intakes*. Using the Tolerable Upper Intake Level for Nutrient Assessment of Groups.

6. FDA. Title 21: Food and Drugs: Part 355: Anticaries Drug Products for Over-the-Counter Human Use. Subpart C Labeling. Revised April 1, 2017

7. American Dental Association Council on Scientific Affairs. Fluoride toothpaste use for young children. *JADA* 145(2):91. February 2014.

8. National Scientific Council on the Developing Child. Early exposure to toxic substances damages brain architecture: Working Paper No. 4. 2006.

9. Kalisinska E et al. Fluoride concentrations in the pineal gland, brain and bone of goosander... *Environ Geochem Health*. 2014; 36:1063-77. Table 1.

Appendix B

Fluoride Research Needed:
National Research Council (2006)

Neurotoxicity and Neurobehavioral Effects
• On the basis of information largely derived from histological, chemical, and molecular studies, <u>it is apparent that fluorides have the ability to interfere with the functions of the brain and the body by direct and indirect means</u>. To determine the possible adverse effects of fluoride, additional data from both the experimental and the clinical sciences are needed.

• The possibility has been raised by the studies conducted in China that <u>fluoride can lower intellectual abilities</u>. Thus, studies of populations exposed to different concentrations of fluoride in drinking water should include measurements of reasoning ability, problem solving, IQ, and short-and long-term memory... Evaluate neurochemical changes that may be associated with dementia.

• Additional animal studies designed to evaluate reasoning are needed. These studies must be carefully designed to measure cognitive skills beyond rote learning or the acquisition of simple associations, and test environmentally relevant doses of fluoride.

• Most of the studies dealing with neural and behavioral responses have tested NaF. It is important to determine whether other forms of fluoride produce the same effects in animal models.

Effects on the Endocrine System
• The inverse correlation between asymptomatic <u>hypothyroidism in pregnant mothers and the IQ of the offspring is a cause for concern</u>. The recent decline in iodine intake in the United States could contribute to increased toxicity of fluoride for some individuals.

• Fluoride is likely to cause decreased melatonin production and to have other effects on normal pineal function, which in turn could contribute to a variety of effects in humans.

Renal and Hepatic Effects
• The effect of low doses of fluoride on kidney and liver enzyme functions in humans needs to be carefully documented in communities exposed to different concentrations of fluoride in drinking water.

Genotoxicity and Carcinogenicity
• Fluoride appears to have the potential to initiate or promote cancers, particularly of the bone.

• In vivo human genotoxicity studies in U.S. populations or other populations with nutritional and sociodemographic variables similar to those in the United States should be conducted.

Measures of Exposure to Fluoride in the United States
• Fluoride should be included in nationwide biomonitoring surveys and nutritional studies. In particular, <u>analysis of fluoride in blood and urine samples taken in these surveys</u> would be valuable.

• To assist in estimating individual fluoride exposure from ingestion, <u>manufacturers and producers should provide information on the fluoride content of commercial foods and beverages</u>.

• Better characterization of exposure to fluoride is needed in epidemiology studies investigating potential effects. Important exposure aspects of such studies would include collecting data on general dietary status and dietary factors that could influence exposure or effects, such as calcium, iodine, and aluminum intakes.

• Characterizing individuals by <u>estimated total exposure,</u> rather than by source of exposure, location of residence, fluoride concentration in drinking water.

> National Research Council. *Fluoride in drinking water: A scientific review of EPA's standards.* National Academies Press; 2006.

A decade after these recommendations were made by the NRC, the only human research done was a major study funded by the National Institute of Environmental Health Sciences. Published in 2017, it found a strong correlation between fluoride levels currently experienced by pregnant women in the US and lower IQ in their children. (See page 56.)

> As discussed in Chapter 1, prenatal fluoride is a major risk factor for preterm birth, and children born preterm are more likely to have lower IQs (page 21).

Appendix C

Fluoridation Chemicals Leach Lead into Drinking Water

Ben Franklin wrote to a colleague about a case of lead poisoning in Europe, wherein a whole family was afflicted by drinking rain water from their leaded roof: "This had been drunk several years without mischief; but some young trees planted near the house growing up above the roof, and shedding the leaves upon it, it was supposed that an acid in those leaves had corroded the lead they covered and furnished the water of that with its baneful particles and qualities."

This problem Franklin described in 1786 is being repeated in our time. Caustic chemicals added to modern tap water are leaching lead from brass plumbing fixtures. Water enters most homes through brass water meters and back-flow valves, travels through brass elbows and shutoff valves, then flows out of brass faucets. Brass contains lead.

Disinfection and fluoridation chemicals have been added to the tap water that hundreds of millions of Americans have been drinking their entire lives. Unbelievable as it seems for a society that prides itself on science, no one had looked at brass corrosion caused by combinations of these corrosive chemicals prior to a landmark 2007 study by the nonprofit Environmental Quality Institute at the University of North Carolina in Asheville.

The researchers of this well-designed study found that when the chemical most often used to fluoridate drinking water is combined with chlorination chemicals, it worsens the leaching of lead from brass elbows and brass water meters.

> "Over the first test week... lead concentrations nearly doubled (from about 100 ppb [parts per billion] to nearly 200), but when fluosilicic acid was also included, lead concentrations spiked to over 900 ppb. Fluosilicic acid, the most widely used fluoridating agent, is a good solvent for lead. Lead concentrations from the chlorine-based waters decreased over the study period, while for the chloramines + ammonia + fluosilicic acid combination, lead concentrations increased with time."[1]

In communities where fluosilicic acid is added to drinking water, the prevalence of children with blood-lead levels over 10 micrograms per deciliter is about double that in nonfluoridated communities.[2]

Evidence of Lead Leaching into Fluoridated Drinking Water

Several cities have discovered that increased lead levels in their drinking water was caused by the fluoridation chemicals. When Tacoma, Washington had to shut down fluoridation in 1992, lead levels in water dropped from 32 to 17 ppb. After the equipment was fixed, the lead levels shot right back up to 32 ppb. The city discontinued the use of fluoride, and the lead levels again dropped.[3]

Thurmont, Maryland's lead levels decreased significantly after officials stopped adding fluoride. Residents then voted in 1994 to ban fluoridation of their drinking water.[4]

Lebanon, Oregon's tap water contained more lead after fluoridation began in 2001. The City Administrator said that fluoride changed the water chemistry enough to cause more lead to be leached from pipes in older homes.[5]

When New York City's fluoridation treatment was shut down for 3 to 4 months, there was approximately a 20% decrease in the lead concentration in city water.[6]

Fluosilicic acid leaches copper from brass plumbing into drinking water. Copper is a recently recognized risk factor for Alzheimer's disease, whose death rates are 25% higher in the most fluoridated states. (See page 74.)

From "Overdosed: Fluoride, Copper, and Alzheimer's Disease,"
the author's report published in the Oct. 2013 *Townsend Letter*.
Linked from: PregnancyAndFluorideDoNotMix.com/author

References

1. Maas RP, Patch SC, Christian AM, Coplan MJ. Effects of fluoridation and disinfection agent combinations on lead leaching from leaded-brass parts. *Neurotoxicology*. Sep 2007;28(5):1023–1031.

2. Coplan MJ, Patch SC, Masters RD, Bachman MS. Confirmation of and explanations for elevated blood lead and other disorders in children exposed to water disinfection and fluoridation chemicals. *Neurotoxicology* 2007 Sep; 28(5):1032–1042.

3. Tacoma Public Utilities. Letter to Department of Health. Dec. 2, 1992.

4. Lead levels in Thurmont water drop. *The Frederick Post*. Feb. 3, 1994.

5. Fluoride bill has no effect on cities in the mid-valley. *Albany Democrat-Herald*. Feb. 24, 2005.

6. Personal communication. Environmental Quality Institute. Feb. 6, 2008.

Appendix D

Why We Should Not Believe the Fluoridation Sales Pitch

Fluoridation promoters are obsessed with decayed teeth, to a 100th of a tooth surface. They avoid mentioning healthy teeth, and for good reason: it blows away their house of cards. A major Australian survey, however, did report the total number of teeth, which for 12-year olds is 24 teeth.

In fluoridated areas, 12-year olds averaged about one tooth that was "decayed, missing, or filled" (past or present decay). In unfluoridated areas, it was about 1½ teeth. That ½-tooth difference, the authors say is a "relative difference" of 50% more decay.[1] True, but relative percentages are extremely deceptive, as the actual numbers prove:

> Out of 24 total teeth, unfluoridated 12-year olds averaged 22.5 and fluoridated ones 23 healthy teeth. That ½-tooth is only a **2% difference in healthy teeth**.

One of the authors repeated the same deception 8 years later. For 12-year olds, less than a ½-tooth (0.44) was a 51% relative difference in decayed teeth. Although only a **2% difference in healthy teeth**, this fluoride salesman claimed it was "considerable evidence regarding the effectiveness of water fluoridation at an individual level."[2]

US Government's Best Evidence for Fluoridation
This major study compared the number of tooth <u>surfaces</u> that were decayed, missing, or filled in the permanent teeth of 39,000 children. For 12-year olds, the difference was <u>½ of one tooth surface</u>.[3]

> A tooth has 4 or 5 surfaces, so 12-year olds (24 teeth) have at least 100 tooth surfaces. A ½ surface is only **0.5% difference in healthy teeth** – in <u>oral health</u> – the reason for fluoridation.

The difference for all ages (5-17 years old) also averaged about <u>½ of a surface</u> (3.39 vs 2.79 decayed tooth surfaces). But the government dentists claimed a relative difference (0.6 ÷ 3.39) of 18% less decay, and fluoridation promoters have used that deception for decades to convince us of the dire need to inject fluoride into our drinking water.

2018 – It Gets Worse
Because there is a "<u>paucity</u> of studies" for the effectiveness of fluoridation, promoters calculated the number of decayed permanent teeth in 12,604 children and adolescents (1999-2004 and 2011-2014).

After adjustments (for age, sex, race/ethnicity, rural-urban location, head-of-household education, and period since last dental visit), the difference in decay attributed to fluoridated water was a negligible three-tenths of one tooth surface – **0.3% difference in oral health** – but the fluoridation promoters called this a "statistically significant... substantial caries-preventive benefit" for US children.[4]

Don't Be Takin' Fluoride
Many people, including health professionals, continue to buy this nonsense. If you do, ask yourself why you believe this. What do you actually know about fluoridation, beyond its deceptive sales pitch?

An analogy: on Diet A, the weight of obese young children decreased by 5 pounds (from an average of 100 to 95). On Diet B, it decreased one pound more to 94 pounds, a 1% decrease in final weight. Would you buy the sales pitch: "Diet B Increases Weight Loss by 20%"?

"Half the truth is often a great lie." – Benjamin Franklin

FDA Confirms Ineffectiveness of Drinking Fluoridated Water
Based on the best evidence submitted by fluoridation promoters, the FDA would not allow a claim suggesting 50% less, nor even 1% less tooth decay. Instead, only this vague feeble health claim is permitted:

"Drinking fluoridated water may reduce the risk of tooth decay."[5]

May reduce risk? The same can be said for drinking pure water.

References

1. Armfield JM, Slade GD, Spencer AJ. Water fluoridation and children's dental health. The Child Dental Health Survey, Australia 2002. Page 28. Dental Statistics and Research Series Number 36.

2. Armfield JM. Community effectiveness of public water fluoridation in reducing children's dental disease. *Public Health Rep.* 2010 Sep-Oct; 125(5);655–664.

3. Brunelle JA, Carlos JP. Recent trends in dental caries in U.S. children and the effect of water fluoridation. *J Dent Res.* 1990 Feb;69(Special Issue):723–727.

4. Slade GD, Grider WB, Maas WR, Sanders AE. Water fluoridation and dental caries in U.S. children and adolescents. *J Dent Res.* 2018 May 1:22034518774331.

5. Food and Drug Administration. Health claim notification for fluoridated water and reduced risk of dental caries. 2006.

I've had the pleasure of knowing John D. MacArthur for 20 years. During that time, I've watched him take on complex research, going deep into the origin of ideas and not quitting until he's satisfied that the search has been as fruitful as he could possibly muster at that time. Following that effort, he's been able to see where others have left out necessary lines of inquiry. John has taken hold of those overlooked areas to research and write, backfilling the knowledge vacuums in an effort to make human understandings more complete.

– Michael Diamond

Michael Diamond has long championed the US Constitution's *Domestic Violence Clause*, the overlooked provision the Founders gave us that obligates and empowers Americans to protect one another from unforeseen harms that we would bring upon ourselves. (DomesticViolenceClause.org)

Also by the author

Mind Over Gray Matter:
Practical Neuroscience
from the Decade of the Brain

Know Your Brain

This book is all about your brain –
the nourishment it needs, the exercise it craves,
the rest it requires, the protection it deserves –
practical neuroscience you can use for the
best performance of your life.

FEED and NOURISH your brain, so you can survive and thrive.
The Brain-Food Pyramid's four sides represent the dietary elements
that construct and connect, power and protect your brain.

STIMULATE and EXERCISE your brain, so you can learn and excel.
Your brain needs mental stimulation and the benefits of physical
exercise to function optimally and make new connections throughout life.

DE-STRESS and REST your brain, so you can relax and recharge.
Stress has very real effects on your brain's ability to remember and learn.
Cultivating your relaxation response will maintain your mental well-being.

SAFEGUARD and PROTECT your brain, so you can live long and prosper.
Your brain is vulnerable to physical trauma and chemical toxins
that can compromise your cognitive ability and human potential.

Enrich Your Life

Mind Over Gray Matter includes the numerous
reports that John wrote for the Franklin Institute
Science Museum's comprehensive online
resource (2001 to 2007): "The Human Brain."

27384813R00054

Made in the USA
Columbia, SC
26 September 2018